Breast Calcification
A Diagnostic Manual

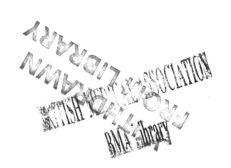

Breast Calcification
A Diagnostic Manual

Edited by

Andy Evans
Consultant Radiologist
Breast Services
International Breast Education Centre
City Hospital, Hucknall Road
Nottingham, UK

Ian Ellis
Reader and Consultant in Pathology
Department of Histopathology
City Hospital, Hucknall Road
Nottingham, UK

Sarah Pinder
Senior Lecturer in Histopathology
Department of Histopathology
City Hospital, Hucknall Road
Nottingham, UK

Robin Wilson
Consultant Radiologist
International Breast Education Centre
City Hospital, Hucknall Road
Nottingham, UK

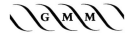

Greenwich Medical Media
4th Floor, 137 Euston Road
London
NW1 2AA

870 Market Street, Ste 720
San Francisco
CA 94109, USA

ISBN number 1841101117

First Published 2002

Distributed worldwide by Plymbridge Distributors Ltd and in the USA by Jamco

Typeset by Phoenix Photosetting, Chatham, Kent

Printed by MPG Books Ltd, Bodmin, Cornwall

**Visit our website at
www.greenwich-medical.co.uk**

Contents

Preface

Breast calcification seen on mammography often represents difficult and complex diagnostic challenges. Calcifications are more difficult to detect, analyse and biopsy than other mammographic abnormalities. There has been a great deal of research and technical advances in this area over the last 10 years. Despite this, the value of detecting breast calcification remains controversial and the continued subject of debate amongst breast radiologists, pathologists and clinicians.

Current practice means that some women are harmed by the detection of mammographic calcification by being subjected to a variety of investigations ranging from recall for magnification views to surgical localisation biopsy for what proves to be benign disease or normality.

Although current percutaneous biopsy techniques have reduced the number of women undergoing surgical biopsy for benign calcifications, the process of recall, further views, percutaneous biopsy and return for results is stressful. Most calcifications recalled at screening are benign and their detection and investigation confers no benefit.

Mammographic calcification is, however, an important feature of invasive and in situ breast cancer. Its detection enables the diagnosis of high-grade invasive cancer at small sizes when the prognosis is good. The detection of high-grade DCIS prevents the development of high-grade invasive breast cancer and so saves lives. The value of diagnosing low-grade DCIS is less clear as a significant proportion of these lesions would never have become invasive in the woman's lifetime.

This book brings together in one volume, current thinking on the detection and diagnosis of breast calcification. Current issues such as computer-aided detection, choice of biopsy technique, assessing adequacy of percutaneous biopsy, predicting and diagnosing invasion will be addressed as well as more novel approaches and ideas, such as the use of synchrotron radiation for diagnosis and the use of mammographic calcification as a prognostic factor.

We hope this book will help those involved in managing women with breast calcification to re-evaluate their own methods of detection and diagnosis, the value of detecting such calcification and where the future lies in this fascinating field.

Andy Evans May 2002

Contributors

Sue Astley
Imaging Science and Biomedical
Engineering
University of Manchester
Stopford Building
Oxford Road
Manchester, UK

Helen Burrell
Department of Radiology
Breast Screening Unit
City Hospital
Hucknall Road
Nottingham, UK

Fiona Gilbert
Academic Department of Radiology
University of Aberdeen
West Block, Polwarth Building
Foresterhill
Aberdeen, UK

Robert A Lewis
School of Physics and Materials Engineering
Monash University
Victoria
Australia

Douglas McMillan
Professorial Unit of Surgery
City Hospital
Hucknall Road
Nottingham, UK

Keith D Rodgers
Department of Materials and Medical
Services
Cranfield University
Shrivenham
Swindon
Wiltshire , UK

Will L Teh
Department of Radiology
Northwick Park and St Marks Hospital
Watford Road
Harrow, UK

Acknowledgement

I would like to thank Joanne Cooper who despite working tirelessly preparing the manuscript and organising the book has remained helpful and cheerful.

Breast benign calcification

Andy Evans and Ian Ellis

Introduction

Calcification is the mammographic feature most commonly associated with benign, screening-provoked surgical biopsy[1]. The widespread introduction of image-guided core biopsy and digital stereotaxis has made the non-operative diagnosis of indeterminate mammographic calcification easier and more reliable. A consecutive series of 174 benign, screen-detected calcification clusters suspicious enough to warrant biopsy indicates that 87% of such calcification clusters were able to be confidently diagnosed on core

biopsy alone. As can be seen from Table 1.1, the commonest causes of benign indeterminate calcification are fibrocystic change, fibroadenoma, stromal calcification and fibroadenomatoid hyperplasia. Less common causes include involutional change, sclerosing adenosis, duct ectasia, aprocrine change, mucocele and blunt duct adenosis. It is interesting to note that 12% of benign indeterminate mammographic calcification diagnosed on core biopsy have associated usual hyperplasia. This is most commonly found in association with fibrocystic change. Table 1.2 shows benign causes of

Table 1.1 Causes of indeterminate calcification diagnosed by core biopsy alone (*n* = 151)

Pathology	Number (%)	Usual hyperplasia no. (%)
Fibrocystic change	50 (33)	11 (22)
Fibroadenoma	27 (18)	0
Stromal calcification	23 (15)	2 (9)
Fibroadenomatoid hyperplasia	22 (15)	0
Involutional change	17 (11)	1 (6)
Sclerosing adenosis	11 (7)	2 (18)
Duct ectasia	6 (4)	1 (17)
Apocrine change	6 (4)	1 (25)
Blunt duct adenosis	4 (3)	1 (25)
Mucocele	3 (2)	0
Vascular	2 (1)	0
Fat necrosis	2 (1)	0
LCIS	1 (0.6)	0
Radiation change	1 (0.6)	0
Foreign body reaction	1 (0.6)	0

Table 1.2 Causes of indeterminate calcification diagnosed at surgery (*n* = 23)

Pathology	Number (%)
Fibrocystic change	10
Atypical lobular hyperplasia	6
Atypical ductal hyperplasia	4
Papillary lesion	3
Radial scar	1
Duct ectasia	1
Sclerosing	1
Fibroadenoma	1

indeterminate calcification diagnosed at surgical biopsy. In this group almost 50% of such lesions contain atypical hyperplasia of either ductal or lobular type. Usual type hyperplasia is present in over 50%. This group also contains lesions deemed to be of uncertain malignant potential such as papillary lesions and radial scars on the diagnostic core biopsy[2]. In the past, the commonest cause for diagnostic surgery for calcifications was the inability of the radiologist to adequately sample the lesion. With the advent of digital stereotaxis, the commonest reason for surgical biopsy of benign calcifications is of uncertain unalignant potential such as atypical hyperplasia, other forms of epithelial atypia, papillary lesions or radial scar diagnosed on image-guided core biopsy.

Fibrocystic change

Fibrocystic change describes a variety of morphological alterations believed to be an exaggerated response to physiological changes in breast tissue. Symptomatic presentation usually occurs before the menopause as benign appearing masses due to cysts. Symptoms can persist if women go on to hormone replacement therapy in the postmenopausal period. Microscopically, the lining of the cysts found in fibrocystic change are of two types, those lined by cuboidal luminal or attenuated epithelium and those lined by apocrine type epithelium. Calcification when present usually occurs within the cyst fluid (Fig. 1.1).

Calcifications due to fibrocystic change are extremely common and are the commonest cause of benign, indeterminate mammographic calcifications. Many cases of calcification due to fibrocystic change are characteristic enough not to require recall. These cases often demonstrate bilateral diffuse calcification, although the extent of calcification is often asymmetric. Such calcifications often show a multiple lobular distribution and are often much easier to see on the mediolateral oblique view than the CC view (Fig. 1.2). This is because the calcifications lie within small microcysts and the calcific fluid layers out giving a partial "tea cup" appearance on the mediolateral oblique

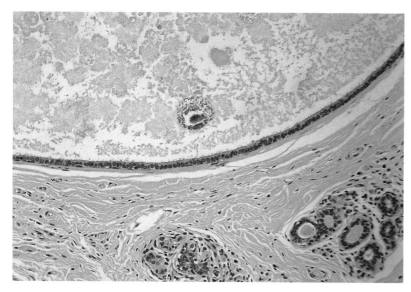

Fig. 1.1
Histology of calcification within cyst fluid.

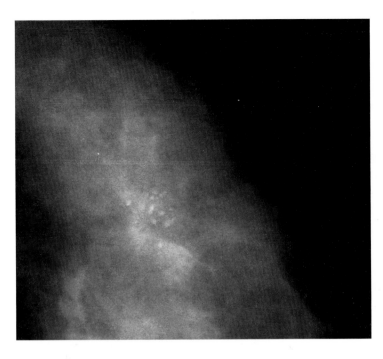

Fig. 1.2
CC view showing low-density rounded calcifications with ill-defined edges due to fibrocystic change.

view but amorphous, low-density, rounded calcifications on the CC view. When a cluster of calcification is due to fibrocystic change, careful inspection of the opposite breast often reveals fainter but similar morphology calcifications. This can often be helpful in preventing recall of benign calcification. Fibrocystic change does, however, commonly present with a single clustered area of granular microcalcifications which show variation in size, density and shape and, as such, are indistinguishable on routine mammographic views from ductal carcinoma in situ (DCIS, Fig. 1.3).

Magnification views are often helpful in demonstrating the tea cup appearance on the lateral magnification view (Fig. 1.4) but many cases of fibrocystic change do not convincingly show this appearance and therefore require image-guided core biopsy. Magnification views of fibrocystic change also commonly demonstrate similar calcifica-

tions elsewhere within the breast. This phenomenon does not, however, exclude the presence of DCIS. Because fibrocystic change is so common, it commonly co-exists with the presence of DCIS. Therefore the presence of one or two tea cups should not preclude image-guided biopsy if some of the other calcifications within the cluster show features highly suspicious of DCIS.

Fibroadenoma and fibroadenomatoid hyperplasia

Fibroadenomas are the commonest cause of a breast lump in the female population. They most commonly occur in women in their 20s and 30s. Calcification within fibroadenomas in women of this age is unusual. After the menopause, fibroadenomas can become hyalanised and suspicious microcalcification

5

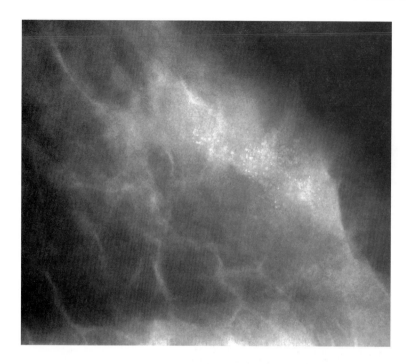

Fig. 1.3
Mammographic image showing an irregularly shaped cluster of pleomorphic calcifications. This area of fibrocystic change was mammographically indistinguishable from DCIS.

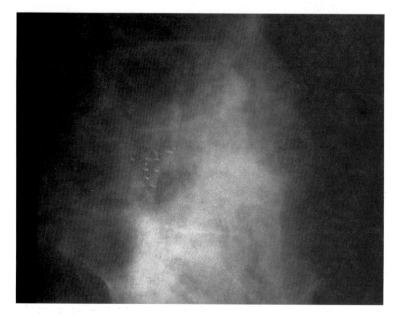

Fig. 1.4
Lateral magnification view of microcalcifications demonstrating the "tea cup" sign indicating fibrocystic change.

can occur which is of dystrophic type and occurs within the stroma or the epithelial clefts (Fig. 1.5).

On mammography coarse, popcorn-like calcifications are often seen in involuting fibroadenomas (Fig. 1.6). Calcification with this characteristic morphology is no cause for concern and does not require recall. Fine calcification can, however, occur within fibroadenomas and, if a dense background

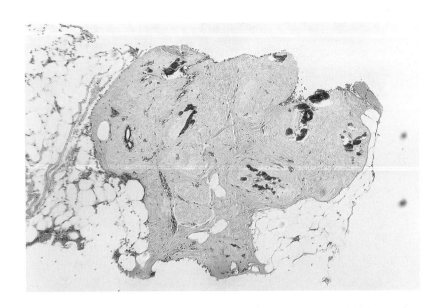

Fig. 1.5
Histological image of dystrophic calcification within fibroadenoma.

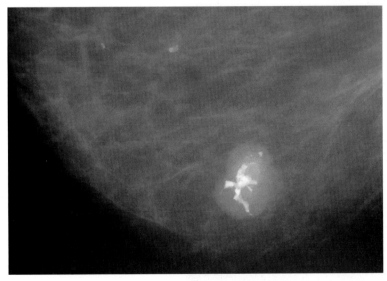

Fig. 1.6
Mammographic image showing coarse popcorn-like calcification within a fibroadenoma.

pattern obscures the well-defined margins of the mass component of the fibroadenoma, such calcifications can cause diagnostic difficulty (Fig. 1.7) and confirmation of their benign nature with image-guided core biopsy is required.

Fibroadenomatoid hyperplasia is a common cause of impalpable mammographic calcification, although it has only been recently described as a cause of suspicious microcalcification[3]. Fibroadenomatoid hyperplasia histologically displays composite features of fibroadenoma and fibrocystic change. Like many benign conditions of the breast it has been previously described under a number of different names, including sclerosing lobular hyperplasia, fibroadenomatosis or fibroadenomatoid mastopathy. It is characterised by a proliferation of fibrous stroma within which are hyperplastic epithe-

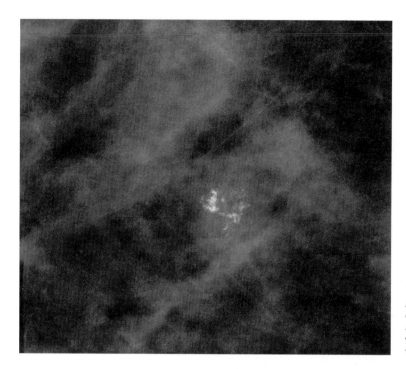

Fig. 1.7
An indeterminate cluster of calcification with no apparent associated mass. Histologically, this was due to calcification within a fibroadenoma.

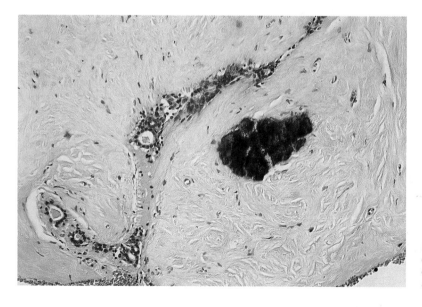

Fig. 1.8
Histological image showing calcification within the stromal component of fibro-adenomatoid hyperplasia.

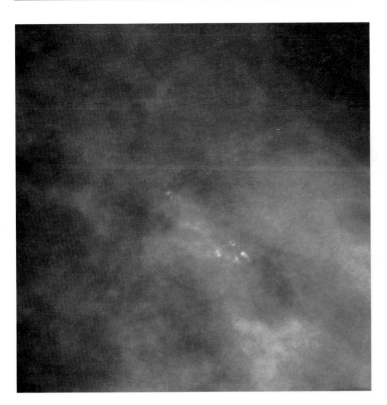

Fig. 1.9
Mammographic image showing irregularly shaped cluster of pleomorphic granular microcalcifications due to fibroadenomatoid hyperplasia.

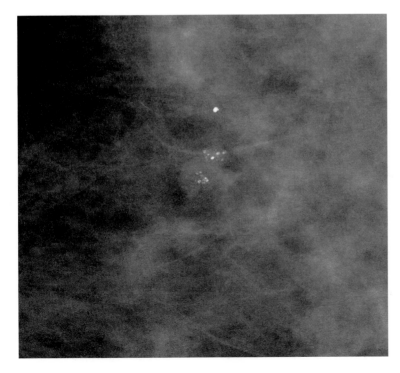

Fig. 1.10
Granular and punctate calcifications varying in size and density due to fibroadenomatoid hyperplasia.

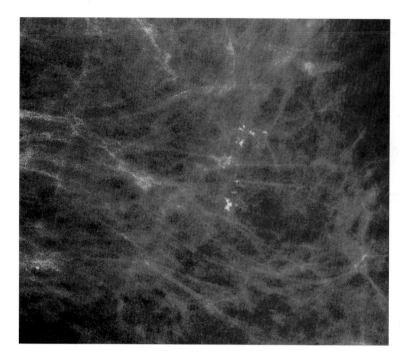

Fig. 1.11
Mammographic image showing a cluster of microcalcification with no associated density. The calcifications contain rod-like forms as well as granular and punctate calcifications. Histologically, this is fibro-adenomatoid hyperplasia.

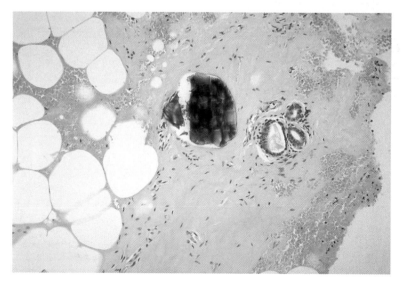

Fig. 1.12
Histological image showing calcification of normal breast stroma.

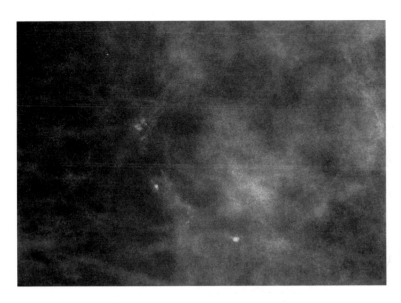

Fig. 1.13
An indeterminate elongated cluster of calcifications containing granular and punctate forms. Histologically, this was due to stromal calcification.

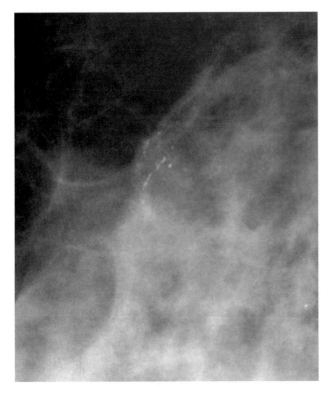

Fig. 1.14
Mammographic image showing elongated linear calcifications within a cluster. Histologically, this was stromal calcification.

11

lial elements. Unlike fibroadenoma, fibroadenomatoid hyperplasia does not present as a well-circumscribed mass. Symptomatically, fibroadenomatoid hyperplasia presents in young women with palpable masses. In such symptomatic women, mammography often shows mass lesions and rarely shows calcification. Fibroadenomatoid hyperplasia does, however, cause suspicious microcalcification in postmenopausal women. Calcification generally occurs following hyaline degeneration of the stromal component (Fig. 1.8).

The radiological features of fibroadenomatoid hyperplasia manifesting as calcification are those of granular microcalcifications that show variation in shape, size and density. It virtually always presents with calcification in a localised, irregularly shaped cluster. Rod-shaped calcifications are common. Branching calcifications and a ductal distribution are seen in a minority of cases (Figs 1.9–1.11). Histologically, the calcifications seen in fibroadenomatoid hyperplasia lie within the stroma in the vast majority of cases and calcification is occasionally seen in the sub-epithelial region. Fibroadenomatoid hyperplasia does not appear to be associated with malignant lesions and it can usually be confidently diagnosed on image-guided core biopsy. Surgical excision is rarely required for diagnostic purposes.

Stromal calcification

Normal breast stroma can occasionally calcify and cause indeterminate mammographic microcalcifications (Fig. 1.12). The calcification clusters vary in size and occasionally can be quite large. In a proportion of cases the calcifications are elongated towards the nipple and this raises a suspicion of DCIS. The calcifications are usually granular in shape and often vary markedly in size and density. Occasionally, elongated rod-like forms are also found. There is usually no associated mammographic density (Figs 1.13 and 1.14).

Calcification within atrophic lobules (involutional change)

Calcification within atrophic lobules can occur (Fig. 1.15) and this can give rise to suspicious microcalcification on mammography. Most cases consist of oval or round clusters of predominantly punctate calcifications but which vary in size and density (Fig. 1.16). Occasionally, however, more suspicious features such as a ductal distribution and elongated linear forms can occur (Figs 1.17 and 1.18).

Sclerosing adenosis

Sclerosing adenosis is an entity composed of a proliferation of epithelial myoepithelial and connective tissue structures within a terminal duct lobular unit. Microscopically, this proliferation of epithelial and interlobular stromal elements results in distortion and expansion of lobules within an overall nodular or diffuse appearance. The epithelial component forms microacinar structures that have small luminal spaces. These luminal spaces frequently contain microcalcification (Fig. 1.19).

Presentation of sclerosing adenosis is varied. Symptomatically, it can often present as a palpable mass that can be ill-defined and fixed, and give a clinical impression of carcinoma. More commonly, sclerosing adenosis presents as a mammographic abnormality. Mammographically, the most common correlate is microcalcification but sclerosing adenosis can also present as areas of parenchymal distortion or an ill-defined mass. Mammographically, the calcifications seen in sclerosing adenosis are always fine and contain a mixture of granular and punctate elements. There is often quite marked variation in size and density of the calcific flecks. The calcifications occur in either round or oval clusters and sometimes a multilobular distribution can be present (Figs

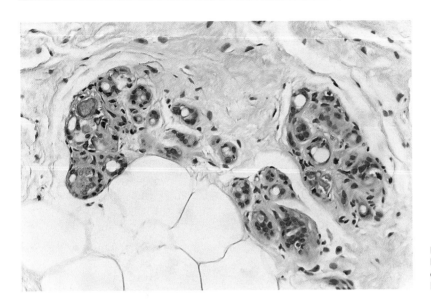

Fig. 1.15
Histological image showing calcification within atrophic lobules.

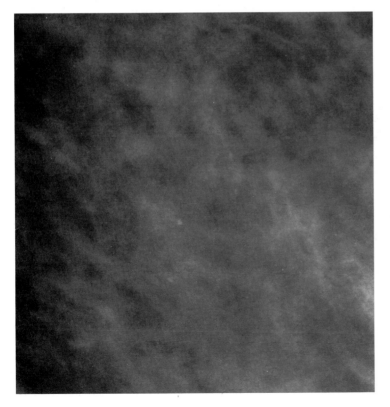

Fig. 1.16
Mammographic image showing predominantly punctate calcifications due to calcification in atrophic lobules.

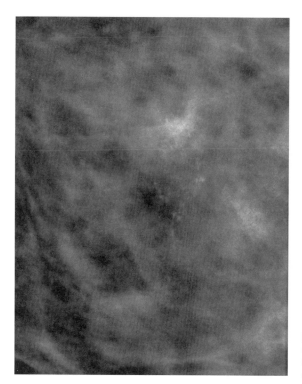

Fig. 1.17
Calcification cluster showing a ductal distribution and elongated rod-shaped forms due to calcification within atrophic lobules.

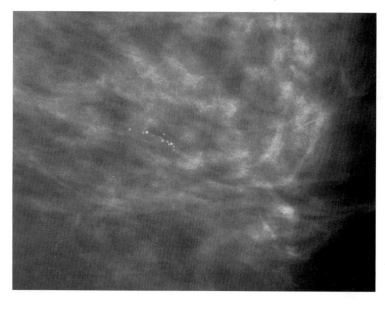

Fig. 1.18
Mammographic image showing granular calcifications with a marked duct distribution due to calcification of atrophic lobules.

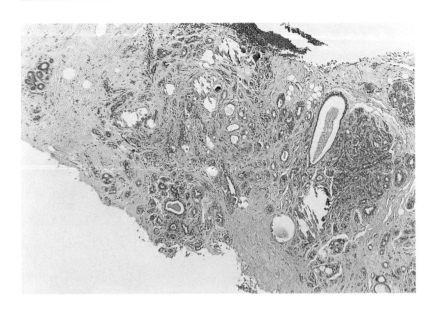

Fig. 1.19
Histological image demonstrating calcification within luminal spaces in sclerosing adenosis.

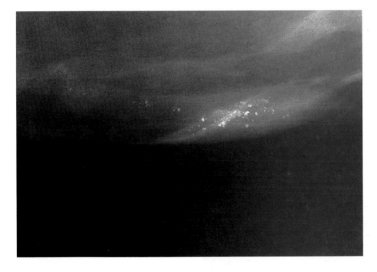

Fig. 1.20
Mammographic image showing an elongated cluster of pleomorphic calcifications due to sclerosing adenosis.

1.20–1.22). Elongated rod and Y shapes and a ductal distribution of calcifications are not usually found.

Duct ectasia

Duct ectasia consists of dilatation of predominantly the sub-areola ducts that are often filled with pultatious material resembling comedo-type DCIS. The duct lining epithelium often contains interspersed inflammatory cells and macrophages. The duct wall and periductal stroma also contain an inflammatory reaction. Duct ectasia is common in smokers, and is often complicated by recurrent periductal abscesses and mammillary

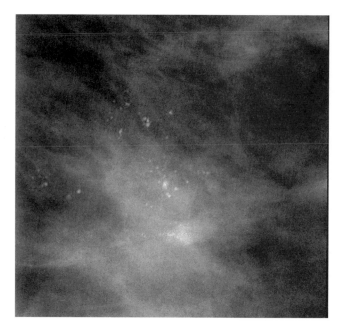

Fig. 1.21
A diffuse cluster of granular and punctate calcifications due to sclerosing adenosis.

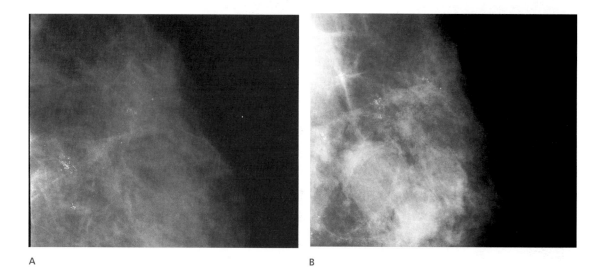

A   B

Fig. 1.22 (A, B)
A widespread microcalcification with a multilobular distribution due to sclerosing adenosis.

fistula. Duct ectasia is also a cause of nipple discharge and nipple retraction. Calcifications due to duct ectasia are often characteristic. The features are those of coarse, rod and branching calcifications in a ductal distribution (Fig. 1.23). These calcifica-tions are formed by calcification of debris within dilated ducts (Fig. 1.24). These intra-ductal calcifications have been described as having a "broken needle appearance". Unlike the ductal calcifications seen in DCIS, it is rare for there to be associated fine granu-

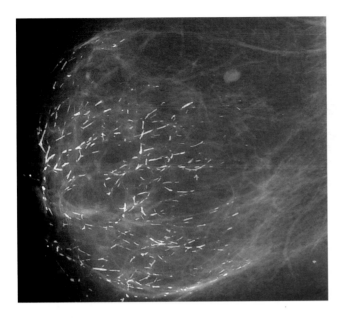

Fig. 1.23
Coarse rod- and branching-shaped calcifications in a ductal distribution due to duct ectasia.

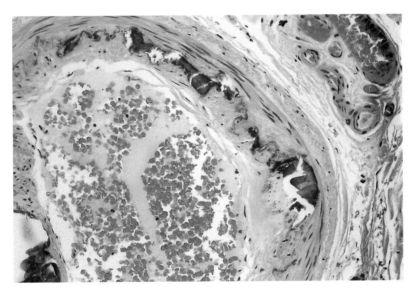

Fig. 1.24
Histological image showing calcification of the wall of a muscular blood vessel.

lar calcifications. In DCIS, although rod and branching calcifications are common, it is very rare for the number of rods and branching calcifications to be higher than the number of fine granular calcifications present. Duct ectasia is very commonly bilateral and this feature is quite useful in confirming the benign nature of small areas of duct ectasia (Fig. 1.25). It is commonly found that

the debris within the duct in duct ectasia extrudes into the surrounding peri-ductal tissues. This causes an inflammatory reaction around the duct. This inflammatory reaction often calcifies, leading to "lead pipe" appearing calcification (Fig 1.26). Very occasionally, high-grade DCIS can produce very coarse calcifications which can be confused with duct ectasia. Caution should therefore be

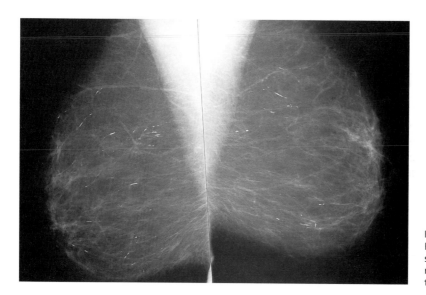

Fig. 1.25
Bilateral mammography showing bilateral widespread rod-shaped calcifications due to duct ectasia.

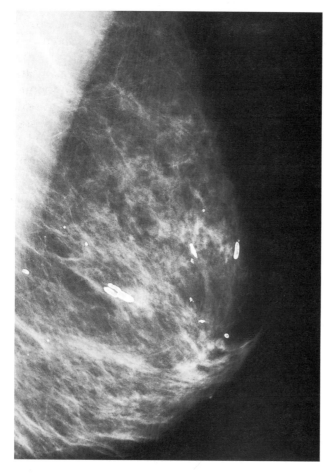

Fig. 1.26
Mammographic image showing lead-pipe calcifications due to calcification of periductal fat necrosis associated with duct ectasia.

exercised in diagnosing a focal, unilateral area of duct ectasia.

Blunt duct adenosis

Blunt duct adenosis is a common condition which forms part of the spectrum of fibrocystic change. It may manifest as a dominant condition but rarely produces a symptomatic lesion in isolation. Microcalcification of luminal secretions can occur and this results in its detection by mammography (Fig. 1.27). Microscopically, blunt duct adenosis is characterised by the replacement of the normal lobular luminal epithelium by a layer of tall columnar epithelial cells with basal nuclei and apical cytoplasmic snouts. No atypia is usually present but nuclei may be enlarged. Mild stromal proliferation can be seen in association with blunt duct adenosis. The columnar cells may secrete mucinous material to form microcysts and calcification of cyst contents can occur[7,8].

Mammographically, blunt duct adenosis is characterised by a small oval or round cluster or granular microcalcification (Fig. 1.28). Linear and rod-shaped forms are usually absent and there is normally no ductal distribution.

Vascular calcification

Vascular calcification is common and is usually not a diagnostic problem. It is characterised by serpentine, tramline calcifications (Fig. 1.29). Magnification views are occasionally helpful in characterising the nature of vascular calcification. On occasion, early vascular calcification can cause diagnostic problems. If only one side of one vessel calcifies within an area of dense breast tissue this can give a false appearance of ductal calcification. We have occasionally inadvertently confirmed vascular calcification within image-guided core biopsy or Mammotome™. The amount of

postprocedure compressions required in such cases is longer than usual!

A large study from The Netherlands (the DOM project) has shown an association between breast arterial calcification and a number of disorders related to increased or accelerated arterial sclerosis; these include hypertension, transient ischaemic attack and stroke and myocardial infarction. In older women there is an increased risk of diabetes[9]. A similar study from the USA, looking at women who have had both mammography and coronary arteriography, did find an association between breast arterial calcification and ischaemic heart disease but only when the women were aged 59 years or less[10].

Fat necrosis

Fat necrosis is a benign non-suppurative inflammatory process that most commonly occurs subsequent to accidental or iatrogenic breast trauma (Fig. 1.30). Clinically, fat necrosis has a multitude of features varying from single or multiple smooth round nodules to fixed irregular masses which simulate malignancy. The mammographic findings of fat necrosis include lipid cysts, microcalcifications (Figs 1.31 and 1.32), coarse calcifications and spiculated masses. Fat necrosis uncommonly causes focally clustered pleomorphic microcalcifications which are indistinguishable from malignancy[11].

Skin calcification

Skin calcification is commonly demonstrated on screening mammograms and they usually show characteristic round calcifications with a lucent centre; these calcifications are often clustered but the individual calcifications are normally of a similar size. Skin calcifications are often bilateral and symmetrical (Figs 1.33–1.35). Very rarely, skin calcification of a different morphology can be seen in systemic

1

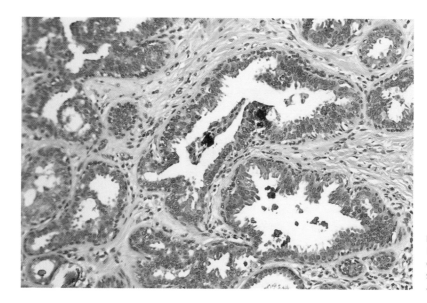

Fig. 1.27
Histological image showing calcification in luminal secretions due to blunt duct adenosis.

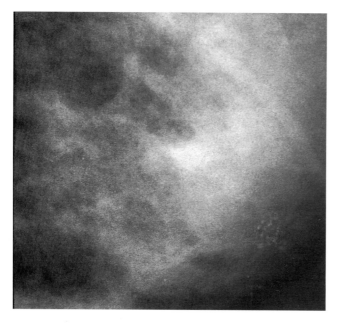

Fig. 1.28
Mammographic image showing a rounded cluster of pleomorphic granular microcalcifications due to blunt duct adenosis.

disorders such as dermatomyositis. Dermatomyositis has been shown to cause bizarre sheet-like branching calcifications[12]. Soft-tissue calcification can occur in this condition between 4 months and 12 years after the onset of the disease. There have been a number of reports of resolution at the calcifications associated with dermatomyositis

using low-dose warfarin treatment. Focal skin lesions commonly calcify and skin papillomas are the commonest cause of abnormal focal skin calcification. Calcified papillomas have an obvious cauliflower morphology and do not normally cause diagnostic difficulties. Occasionally, however, focal skin lesions can cause indeterminate

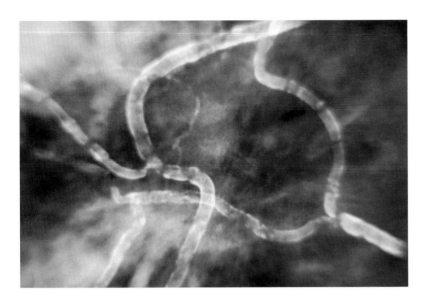

Fig. 1.29
Mammographic image showing serpentine, tram-line calcification characteristic of vascular calcification.

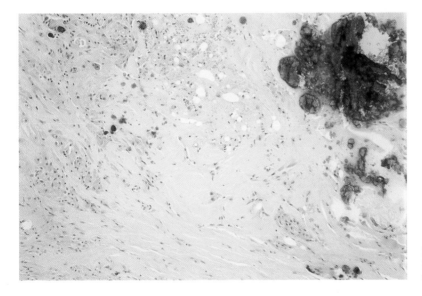

Fig. 1.30
Histological image showing calcification within fat necrosis.

calcification (Fig. 1.36). Their nature can usually be confirmed with tangential views. Occasionally, core biopsy is required.

A number of skin creams, ointments and powders that contain metallic salts can mimic breast calcification. These include deodorants, talcum powder, zinc oxide and gold injections. Soap has also been described as a cause of an artifact that can mimic intra-

mammary breast calcification[13]. Tattoo marks have also been described as simulating intra-mammary calcification.

Suture calcification

Calcification of surgical sutures is occasionally seen, especially in the irradiated breast. The coarse linear morphology of the

21

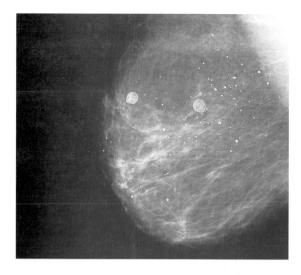

Fig. 1.31
A mammographic image following previous excision of a benign abnormality. Widespread punctate calcifications are demonstrated due to fat necrosis; in addition, calcified oil cysts are seen.

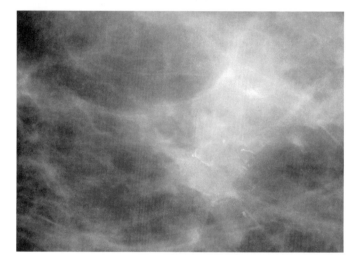

(A)

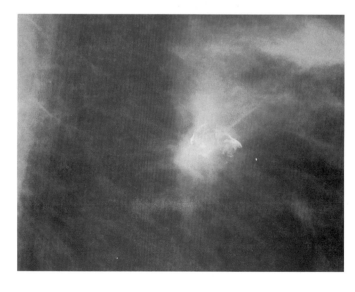

(B)

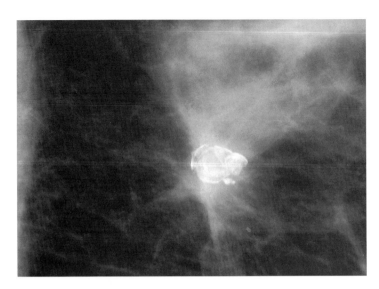

(C)

Fig. 1.32
A series of mammographic images showing the development of calcification due to postoperative fat necrosis. (A) Demonstrates elongated linear calcification which could be viewed as suspicious of malignancy. (B) Illustrates coarsening of the calcification and the development of the characteristic curvilinear calcification seen in fat necrosis. (C) Further coarsening of the calcifications demonstrated the calcification is now obviously benign.

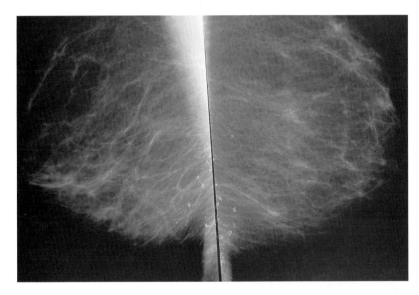

Fig. 1.33
Mammographic image showing skin calcification symmetrically distributed in the inferior breast.

calcifications is usually very characteristic and virtually never causes diagnostic difficulties (Fig. 1.37).

Epidermal inclusion cysts of the breast

Although the characteristic finding of epidermal inclusion cysts are those of a well-circumscribed low-density mass in a subcutaneous location, approximately 30% are associated with heterogeneous microcalcifications[14].

Metastatic calcification due to renal failure

Women with a secondary hyperparathyroid induced by chronic renal failure have

1

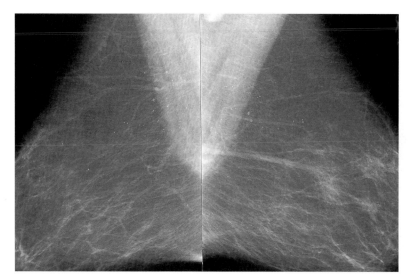

Fig. 1.34
Bilateral mammography showing symmetrically distributed skin calcification adjacent to the pectoral muscle.

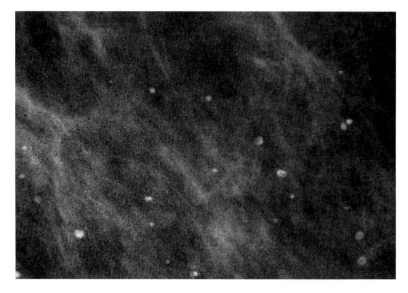

Fig. 1.35
Magnified mammographic image of skin calcification. The characteristic round calcifications with lucent centres is demonstrated.

increased breast calcification. Such calcifications include an increase in vascular and breast parenchymal calcifications. The pattern of such calcification is, however, usually of a benign morphology. Suspicious microcalcification needs to be treated in the same way whether a woman has secondary hyperparathyroidism or not.

Klippel–Trenaunay syndrome

Breast calcification has been reported in association with Klippel–Trenaunay syndrome. The calcification occurred within the subcutaneous adipose tissue due to capillary and small venial proliferation. These contained intramural calcium deposits[15].

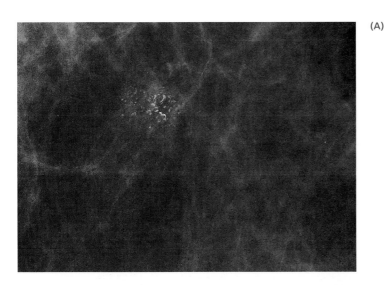

(A)

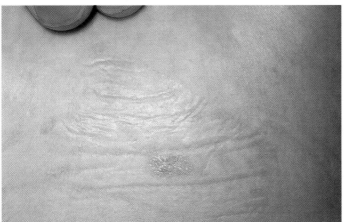

(B)

(C)

Fig. 1.36
(A) Mammographic image of an area of indeterminate calcification for which image-guided core biopsy was planned. (B) The patient volunteered during the prebiopsy consultation that she had a skin lesion which had a similar appearance to the calcification. (C) Mammography following placement of a lead shot over the skin lesion confirmed that the calcification was indeed within the skin.

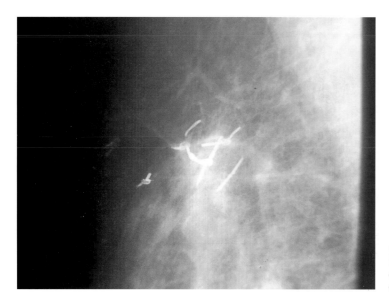

Fig. 1.37
Mammographic image showing the characteristic appearance of suture calcification.

Idiopathic granulomatous mastitis

Granulomatous mastitis occurs in women of reproductive age and usually presents as a tender mass which may be associated with axillary lymphadenopathy and is often bilateral. Microscopic features include a granulomatous inflammatory cell infiltrate centred on, and distorting, lobules.

Mammographic features include areas of coarse dystrophic calcification, which is often multifocal and bilateral (Fig. 1.38). Biopsy is rarely required as the calcification morphology is not usually suspicious of malignancy (Figs 1.39 and 1.40).

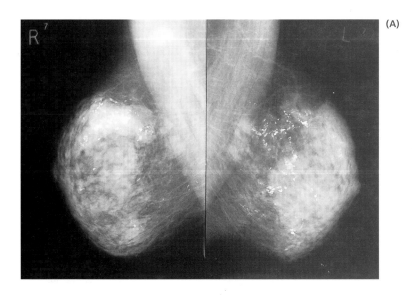

(A)

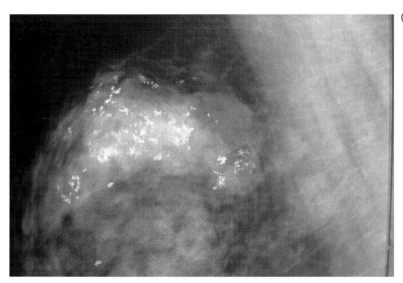

(B)

Fig. 1.38
(A) Bilateral mammography showing bilateral widespread relatively coarse calcifications. (B) A close-up view shows the coarse dystrophic nature of the calcifications with the absence of fine granular calcifications. The appearances are of granulomatous mastitis.

1

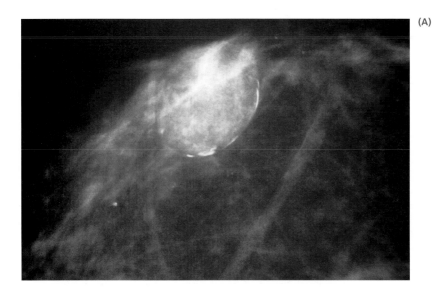

(A)

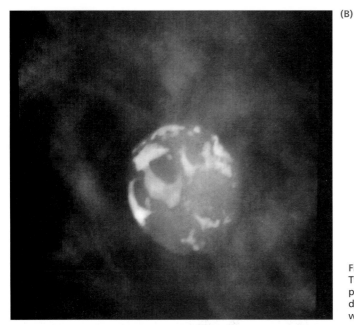

(B)

Fig. 1.39
Two cases showing a well-defined mass with peripheral calcification. Calcification with this distribution is normally found within calcified walls of cysts, oil cysts or haematomas.

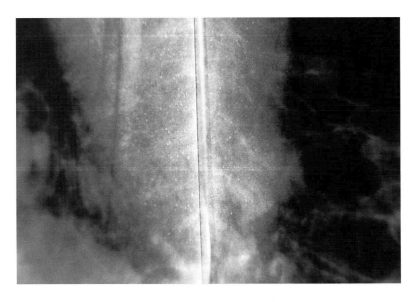

Fig. 1.40
Bilateral mammography shows diffuse punctate calcifications within both pectoral muscles. This is due to previous infection with *Trichinella spiralis*.

References

1. Spencer NJB, Evans AJ, Galea M et al. Pathological–radiological correlations in benign lesions excised during a breast screening programme. Clin Radiol 1994; 49: 853–6.
2. Ellis IO, Humphries S, Michell M, Pinder SE, Wells CA, MDZ Guidelines for non-operative diagnostic procedures and reporting in breast cancer screening: NHSBSP 2001, Report No. 50.
3. Kamal M, Evans AJ, Denley H, Pinder SE, Ellis IO. Fibroadenomatoid hyperplasia: a cause of suspicious microcalcification on screening mammography. Am J Roentgenol 1998; 171: 1331–4.
4. Bundred NJ, Dover MS, Alunwihore N, Faragher EB, Morrison JM. Smoking and peri-ductal mastitis. Br Med J 1993; 307: 772–3.
5. Dixon JM, ed. ABC of Breast Disease. London: BMJ Books, 2001.
6. Hughes LE, Mansell RE, Webster DJT. Benign Disorders and Diseases of the Breast. London: Baillière Tindall, 1989.
7. Chinyama CN, J.D.D. Mammary mucinous lesions; congeners, prevalence and important pathological associations. Histopathology 1996; 29: 533–9.
8. Fraser JL, Raza S, Chorny K, Connolly JL, Schnitt SJ. Columnar alteration with prominent apical snouts and secretions. Am J Surg Pathol 1998; 22: 1521–7.
9. Van Noord PA, Beijerink D, Kemmeren JM, Van der Graaf Y. Mammograms may convey more than breast cancer risk: breast arterial calcification and arterio-sclerotic related disease in women of the DOM cohort. Eur J Cancer Prev 1996; 5: 483–7.
10. Moshyedi AC, Puthwala AH, Kurland RJ, O'Leary DH. Breast arterial calcification: association with coronary artery disease. Radiology 1995; 194: 181–3.
11. Hogge JP, Robinson RE, Magnant CM, Zuurbier RA. The mammographic spectrum of fat necrosis of the breast. Radiographics 1995; 15: 1347–56.
12. Nye PJ, Perrymore WD. Mammographic appearance of calcinosis in dermatomyositis. Am J Roentgenol 1995; 164: 765–6.
13. Thomas DR, Fisher MS, Caroline DF. Case report: soap-author artifact that can mimic intramammary calcifications. Clin Radiol 1995; 50: 64–5.
14. Denison CM, Ward VL, Lester SC et al. Epidermal inclusion cysts of the breasts: three lesions with calcifications. Radiology 1997; 204: 493–6.
15. Apesteguia L, Pina L, Inchusta M et al. Klippel–Trenaunay syndrome: a very infrequent cause of microcalcifications in mammography. Eur Radiol 1997; 7: 123–125.

Intraductal epithelial lesions

Andy Evans and Sarah Pinder

Introduction

Intraductal epithelial proliferations in the breast form a spectrum from usual epithelial hyperplasia (UEH) through atypical ductal hyperplasia (ADH) to DCIS. Whilst UEH is commonly seen as a component of fibrocystic change and is of limited clinical significance, identification of DCIS at breast screening has significant implications. DCIS is composed of a proliferation of cytologically malignant epithelial cells contained within breast parenchymal structures with no evidence of invasion across the duct basement membrane.

Radiology of ductal carcinoma in situ

Frequency of abnormal mammography according to clinical presentation

Microcalcification is the commonest mammographic feature of DCIS and is seen in 80% to 90% of those cases with a mammographic abnormality[1]. However, the proportion of symptomatic DCIS with a mammographic abnormality varies according to the clinical presentation.

It is our experience that virtually all cases of DCIS presenting with single nipple discharge have a mammographic abnormality. In contrast, only about half the women with DCIS presenting as Paget's disease of the nipple have a mammographic lesion[2]. Within the literature there is a huge variation in the reported incidence of mammographic abnormalities in patients with Paget's disease of the nipple ranging from 0 to 100% (Fig. 2.1). The reason why patients with Paget's disease should have such a low incidence of mammographic abnormalities is not clear. The majority of DCIS causing Paget's disease of the nipple is high grade and of solid architecture. Although high grade DCIS is normally associated with necrosis and the presence of calcification this is not often seen in DCIS associated with Paget's disease of the nipple.

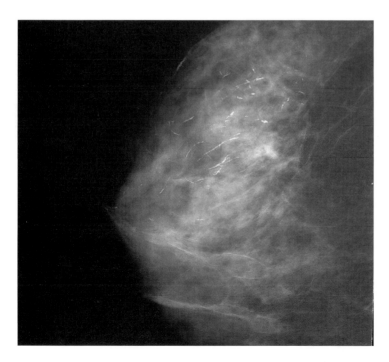

Fig. 2.1
Mammogram showing extensive predominantly linear calcification in a patient with Paget's disease of the nipple. It should be noted how coarse the calcifications are and it is easy for lesions with this appearance to be falsely thought to have duct ectasia.

33

2

DCIS can also present symptomatically as a palpable mass. When it presents in this manner it is more likely to also show a mass lesion mammographically, either entirely solid or a mixed cystic solid lesion when visualised on ultrasound.

DCIS detected by mammographic screening is, by definition, mammographically visible except for the very few lesions picked up due to clinical features noted by radiographers during the screening examination.

Cluster shape

Approximately 80% of cases of calcific DCIS have an irregular cluster shape (Fig. 2.2) and about 10% of these irregular clusters are V-shaped. The irregular cluster shape of DCIS is caused by the growth pattern of DCIS. DCIS has a tendency to grow towards and away from the nipple within a single segment of the breast. About 15% of DCIS clusters have an oval or round cluster shape (Fig. 2.3). DCIS with a round or oval cluster shape is more likely to be confused with benign process than DCIS presenting with an irregular cluster shape. However, the shape of a cluster of calcifications can be particularly helpful when the nature of the individual calcifications are nonspecific. For instance, a round or oval cluster of four or five granular microcalcifications may well be viewed as having a very low risk of being DCIS. A similar number of calcifications within an irregularly shaped cluster (especially if this cluster is elongated towards the nipple) should be viewed with a higher degree of suspicion. Intermediate- and low grade DCIS can present with a multilobular distribution of calcifications where calcifications appear to lie within multiple round or oval clusters within one area of the breast (Fig. 2.4). This distribution which appears to represent disease processes within individual acini of the breast is also commonly found in fibrocystic change.

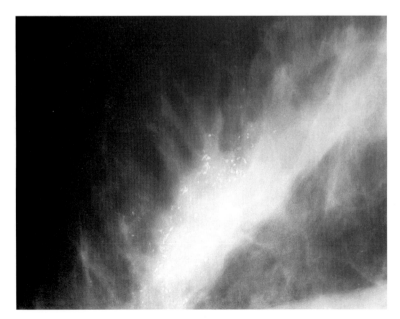

Fig. 2.2
Mammographic view showing an irregularly shaped cluster which is elongated towards the nipple. Histologically, this lesion was high-grade DCIS.

2

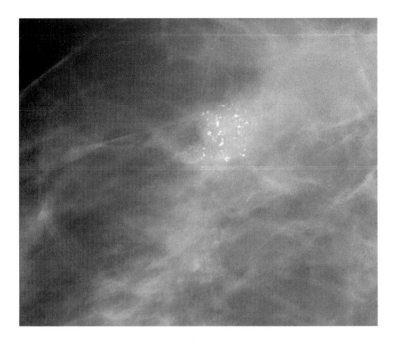

Fig. 2.3
Mammogram showing a rounded cluster of calcifications due to DCIS. The pleomorphism of the granular calcifications thankfully indicated its malignant nature. Pathologically, the lesion was high grade DCIS.

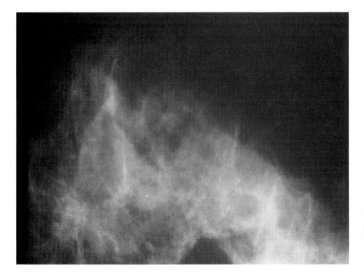

Fig. 2.4
Mammographic view showing a multilobular distribution of calcifications. Such a distribution is commonly found in fibrocystic change but on this occasion was due to intermediate grade DCIS.

Distribution of calcifications in DCIS

One of the commonest and most characteristic features of DCIS is that the calcifications are aligned in a ductal distribution (Fig. 2.5). This distribution is common in both necrotic and non-necrotic DCIS. If calcifications lack rod or branching shapes, a ductal distribution can be extremely helpful in suggesting a malignant cause of the calcifications. The distribution of calcification is also helpful in other ways. Diffuse calcification involving the whole of the breast is unusual and DCIS

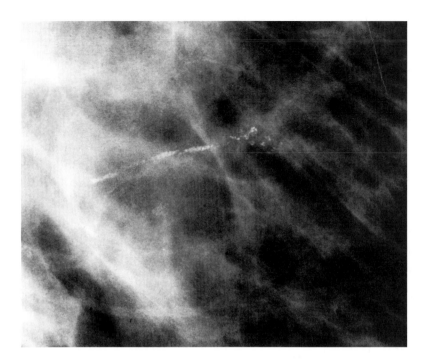

Fig. 2.5
A mammographic image showing inumerable granular microcalcifications in a very obvious ductal distribution. The density of the granular microcalcifications within the duct give it an almost snake skin-like appearance.

of such a large extent will usually also have characteristic calcification features. DCIS is rarely bilateral; diffuse bilateral calcifications are always benign and do not warrant further investigation unless there is a focal area where there is different morphology to the calcifications compared to those elsewhere within the breasts.

The number of calcifications

Approximately 90% of calcification clusters at our unit shown to be DCIS have more than 10 flecks of calcification. However, diagnosing DCIS is not uncommon in lesions with clusters of five or fewer flecks. The decision whether or not to recall three or four flecks of calcification should be made predominantly on the morphology of the calcifications and their distribution and whether the calcifications have changed over time. Recalling patients with mammograms with three flecks

of calcification which are new and in a ductal distribution often leads to a diagnosis of DCIS.

Calcification morphology in DCIS

The most common features of calcifications due to DCIS are granular calcifications with irregularity in density, shape and size compared with the other calcifications within the cluster. Although these features are present in over 90% of cases of DCIS, their usefulness in benign versus malignant differentiation is limited, as these features are also commonly found in benign causes of calcification. The more specific features of DCIS such as a ductal distribution of calcifications, rod and branching shapes are much less common (Fig. 2.6). In our series we found a ductal distribution and rod-

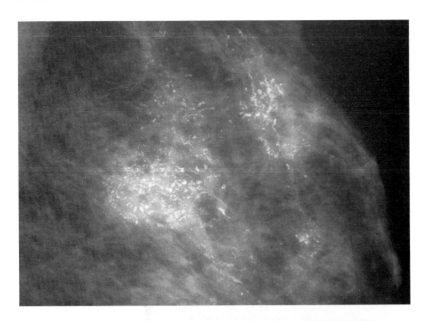

Fig. 2.6
Mammographic image showing a combination of granular, rod and branching calcifications in an irregular cluster distribution. The appearances are pathognomonic of high-grade DCIS.

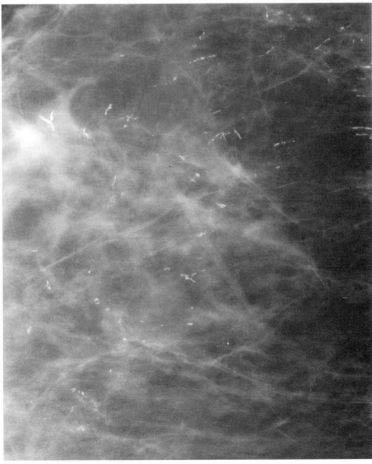

Fig. 2.7
Mammographic image showing quite coarse rod- and Y-shaped calcifications with only a few granular elements. It would be easy to dismiss these calcifications as being due to duct ectasia, in fact they were due to high-grade DCIS with extensive necrosis.

shaped calcifications in about 70% of DCIS cases. Branching calcifications are much less common, being seen in only 40% of cases. The commonest benign cause of branching- and rod-shaped calcifications is duct ectasia and one needs to be particu-larly careful in making a radiological diag-nosis of duct ectasia if the calcifications are unilateral and focal. It is our experience that DCIS presenting as a duct ectasia look-alike is invariably DCIS of high histological grade (Figs 2.7 and 2.8).

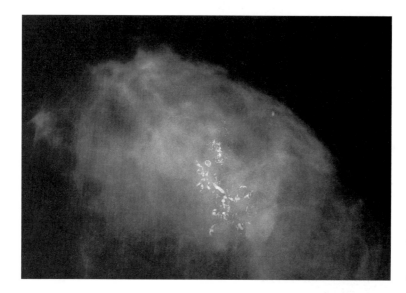

Fig. 2.8
Mammographic image showing a generally coarse cluster of calcifications with predominantly rod and branching calcifications. Histologically, this lesion was high-grade DCIS.

Fig. 2.9
Mammographic image showing a predominantly punctate cluster of microcalcifications in a round cluster shape. It would be easy to dismiss this lesion as benign but it in fact represented low-grade DCIS.

(A)

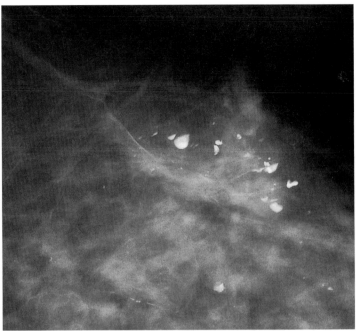

(B)

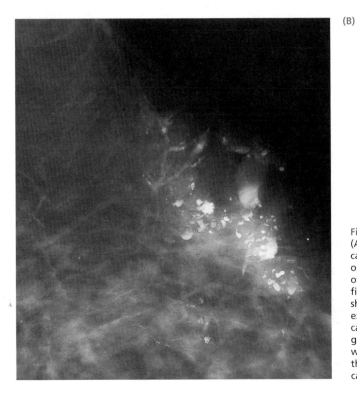

Fig. 2.10
(A) Mammographic image showing coarse calcifications showing definite "tea cupping" on the mediolateral oblique view. The presence of tea cups falsely reassured us that this was fibrocystic change. (B) Taken 3 years later, still shows "tea cupping" but there is now a very extensive ductal branching distribution of the calcification. This was a case of intermediate-grade DCIS with mucin secretion. Calcification within the mucin secretions layered and gave this highly unusual tea cup appearance in this case of DCIS.

Punctate (round or oval) calcifications are also commonly found in DCIS. In our series just under 50% of calcification clusters contained punctate calcifications and about 15% of DCIS calcifications clusters were made up of calcifications which were predominantly punctate in shape (Fig. 2.9). The take-home message is that the presence of relatively benign looking punctate calcifications within a cluster does not exclude DCIS[3].

Changes in the morphology of DCIS calcification over time

A recent study[4] looking at the previous mammograms of women diagnosed as having DCIS showed that in 22% of cases the previous mammograms were, in retrospect, abnormal. This study showed that the following features were commoner on the previous films: predominantly punctate calcification (64% versus 12%, $P = 0.001$) and fewer than 10 calcifications in a cluster (54% versus 24%, $P = 0.05$). Features which were less common on the previous mammogram than the diagnostic mammograms were rod-shaped calcifications (27% versus 64%, $P =$ 0.03) and a ductal distribution of calcifications (45% versus 76%, $P = 0.05$). It can be seen from these results that the calcification morphology of the DCIS present on the previous mammograms are much less characteristic of malignancy than those present at the time of diagnosis. It is also of interest that these cases, which had such non-specific features at the time of previous mammography, were predominantly cases of high grade DCIS. This indicates that the characteristic calcification morphological features of high grade DCIS, i.e. the presence of rods and a ductal distribution may not be present when the lesions are small and that these characteristic features only occur when the lesion grows to larger size (Fig. 2.10A,B). It would therefore be wrong to assume that a small cluster of calcifications containing granular and punctate calcifications represents low grade disease when it is shown to be malignant. Features that were present both on the diagnostic and the previous mammograms, which may have allowed earlier diagnosis, were granular calcifications, which varied in size, density and shape and irregular cluster shape (Fig. 2.11).

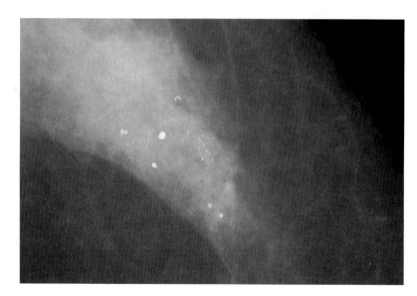

Fig. 2.11
Mammographic image showing a rounded cluster of granular microcalcifications showing slight variation in size, density and shape. This was due to low-grade DCIS.

Growth pattern of calcification due to DCIS

By careful assessment and measurement of mammographic calcification due to DCIS which was missed on previous mammograms and measurement of the site and size of calcification on the later diagnostic images it is possible to gain information concerning DCIS growth rates and growth directions[5]. We have recently found that DCIS grows twice as fast in the nipple plane (i.e. in the plane towards and away from the nipple) as in the plane at 90° to this. However, DCIS appears to grow at equal rates towards and away from the nipple. Apparent DCIS growth at 90° to this nipple plane may just be due to passive expansion of the breast segment. There appears to be a good correlation between both growth in the nipple plane and at 90° to the nipple with the cytonuclear grade of DCIS. This finding supports the validity of current grading systems for DCIS.

The pathological site of mammographic calcifications representing DCIS

Punctate calcifications are commonly found in non-necrotic DCIS. The calcifications are intraductal and occur in intercellular spaces. These spaces are often filled with secretions and it is these that calcify to produce the mammographically visible calcifications in non-necrotic DCIS. Calcifications in the same intercellular spaces may also be granular calcifications. Granular calcifications can, however, be formed in necrotic DCIS as a result of the necrotic debris within the ducts undergoing dystrophic calcification. These granular calcifications can coalesce to form rod-shaped calcifications. If these rod-shaped calcifications occur where the breast duct is branching, then branching calcifications result. Paul Stomper and co-workers

suggested that mammographic calcification may also represent high calcium concentrations within necrotic cells, but presented no direct evidence to confirm this assertion[6].

Appearance of DCIS according to pathological sub-type

Methods for classification are at present under assessment with several groups describing new methods for ascribing histological grade of DCIS. The National Co-ordinating Group for Breast Screening Pathology in the UK recommend a system based on nuclear grade with categories of high, low and intermediate nuclear grade[7]. Support for this classification is provided by the finding that sub-type of DCIS is correlated with the histological grade of the associated invasive tumour; low grade DCIS progresses more often into well-differentiated invasive cancer and high grade DCIS into grade 3 invasive tumour.

High nuclear grade DCIS is composed of pleomorphic large cells with abundant mitoses. The growth pattern is variable and commonly the malignant cells distend the ducts with central calcified necrosis (comedo DCIS) (Fig. 2.12). High-grade DCIS with a cribriform or micropapillary growth pattern may also be seen. DCIS of low nuclear grade is composed of uniform cells with small nuclei. Tumour cell nuclei are hyperchromatic, centrally positioned and have indistinct nucleoli. This sub-type of DCIS most frequently has a cribriform (with geometric "punched out" spaces) or micropapillary pattern (with bulbous projections into the duct lumen). Very often both architectures co-exist, although the cribriform pattern usually predominates (Fig. 2.13). If the neoplastic cells are less pleomorphic than required for the diagnosis of high grade disease but there is a lack of uniformity of low grade DCIS then the lesion is classified as being of intermediate nuclear grade (Fig. 2.14). One or two nucleoli may be seen and are

2

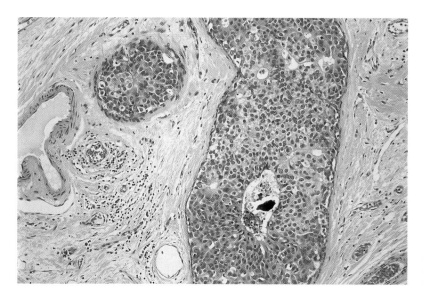

Fig. 2.12
Histological image showing a pleomorphic proliferation of intraductal epithelial cells with central necrosis and calcification. The appearances are of high grade DCIS.

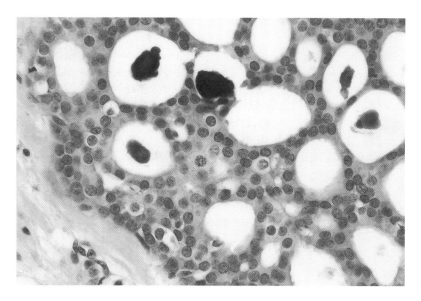

Fig. 2.13
Histological image showing a monotonous intraductal proliferation of epithelial cells. A cribriform architecture is present and there is calcification within the secretions.

more evident than in low nuclear grade DCIS and the nuclear-to-cytoplasmic ratio of tumour cells is often high. As with other grades of DCIS, the architectural pattern may be solid, cribriform or micropapillary. Rarely, variation in the cytonuclear grade of a single DCIS lesion may be seen and then all the nuclear grades present should be recorded but the disease classified according to the highest grade present.

Several other systems for classifying DCIS have been proposed. Some authors have advocated a combined assessment of nuclear grade and necrosis, with high grade, non high-grade with necrosis; and non-high grade without necrosis being recognised[8].

The radiological appearances of DCIS vary markedly according to the pathological sub-type. A variety of molecular markers

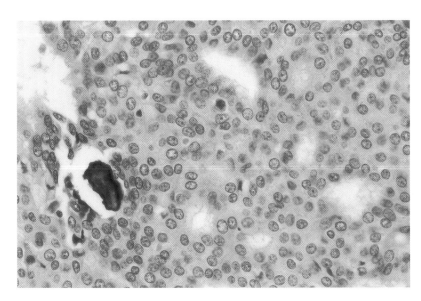

Fig. 2.14
Histological image showing intraductal neoplastic cells less pleomorphic than those of high-grade disease but lacking the uniformity of low-grade DCIS. This is a case of intermediate grade DCIS. Calcification of secretions is again demonstrated.

have also shown a correlation with the radiological features of the disease. The following pathological variables have been shown to correlate with variations in the radiological appearance of DCIS:

- Architectural pattern
- Cell size
- Necrosis
- C-erbB-2 expression
- p53 expression and MIB1
- Oestrogen receptor and progesterone receptor expression

Architectural pattern

The traditional classification of DCIS was based solely on architectural pattern; Holland and co-workers were the first to describe variations in the radiological appearances of DCIS according to architectural pattern[9]. They recorded DCIS cases as either predominantly comedo or predominantly cribriform/micropapillary in architecture and noted that the pathogenesis of the calcification in these sub-types was different. In comedo DCIS, calcification occurs

because of dystrophic calcification within the central necrotic debris, as described above. In cribriform/micropapillary DCIS, however, necrosis is not generally present and it is the secretion in the intercellular spaces which calcifies. The morphology of the calcifications in the two architectural sub-types is also different. Holland et al.[9] found that 80% of the cases of comedo DCIS had linear calcification but this finding was only present in 16% of the cribriform/micropapillary group. This study found that only 53% of the cribriform DCIS group had mammographic calcification compared with 94% of the comedo group. This indicates that calcification in low grade DCIS is variable and often does not occur. Indeed, if calcification does occur, it only occurs within part of the lesion. This paper was also the first to highlight that mammographic estimation of DCIS lesion size was more accurate in comedo DCIS that in the cribriform DCIS. Eight per cent of the comedo and 47% of the cribriform group showed greater than 2 cm discrepancy between mammographic estimation of lesion size and histological measurements[9]. A sub-

2

sequent paper by the same group suggested that by the use of magnification views lesion size estimation in low grade DCIS was as good as lesion size estimation in high grade DCIS[10]. This suggestion was, however, based on a small number of cases and it is difficult to see how magnification views can delineate calcification in areas of low grade DCIS that do not contain histological calcifications. Other authors have confirmed that linear calcifications are more common in the comedo sub-type of DCIS and that granular calcifications are more common in the cribriform/micropapillary types. It is, however, impossible to predict reliably the architectural pattern of DCIS present when only granular calcifications are present. Granular calcifications can be present in both comedo and cribriform DCIS. If there is extensive linear and branching calcification it does, however, indicate a strong likelihood of the presence of high grade DCIS containing necrosis. Modern pathological classifications of DCIS are based on cytonuclear grade alone or in combination with the absence or presence of necrosis.

Cell size

DCIS of large cell size is more likely to display abnormal mammography (94% versus 72%). Calcification is in particular more common in large cell DCIS (95% versus 58%), although comparison of the calcification morphological features of small cell versus large cell DCIS does not show any statistically significant differences. There is, however, a non-significant trend for large cell DCIS to more commonly display a ductal distribution, rod-shaped calcification and an associated asymmetric density. There is a non-significant trend for small cell DCIS calcifications to be predominantly punctate in morphology[1]. The absence of a strong correlation between the cell size and calcification morphology is because not all small cell DCIS is free from necrosis and not all large cell DCIS contains necrosis, and necrosis is the major determinate of calcification morphology in DCIS.

Necrosis

Necrosis within DCIS is an indicator of aggressive biological activity. DCIS with necrosis shows poorer disease-free survival and a higher local recurrence rate compared to DCIS without necrosis. Necrosis has therefore been included as a major determinant in some of the more modern grading systems described for DCIS. As the two mechanisms of calcification formation postulated by Holland et al. are based on the presence or absence of necrosis, it is not surprising that there are strong correlations between the presence or absence of necrosis and the mammographic features of DCIS. DCIS containing necrosis is more likely to show abnormal mammographic findings (95% versus 73%), calcification (96% versus 61%), calcification with a ductal distribution (80% versus 45%) and rod-shaped calcifications (83% versus 45%). DCIS without necrosis is more likely to show abnormal mammographic features without calcification (39% versus 4%) and predominantly punctate calcification (36% versus 13%). The proportion of cases with normal mammograms or abnormal mammograms without calcification appears to show a relationship with both the presence or absence of necrosis and also the degree of necrosis present (Fig. 2.15). The absence of mammographic calcification almost excludes the presence of DCIS with marked necrosis[1].

C-erbB-2 oncogene expression

C-erbB-2 (Her-2, Neu) is a member of the type 1 tyrosine kinase growth factor receptor family. Amplification of c-erbB-2 oncogene and expression of its protein is found in approximately 60% of DCIS cases[11]. C-erbB-2 expression in DCIS has been shown to correlate with aggressive histological features

(A)

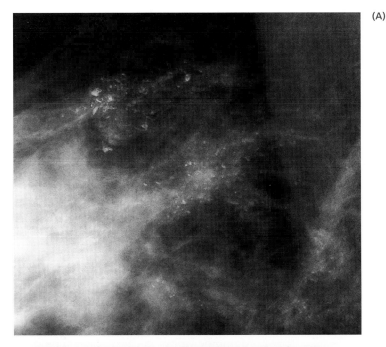

(B)

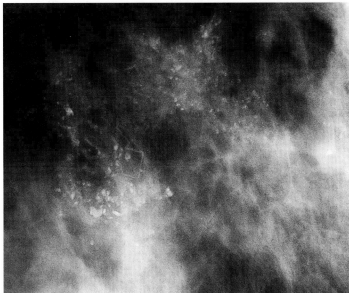

Fig. 2.15
Mammographic images showing a marked branching ductal distribution of calcifications which are, however, of very low density. In this unusual case, the calcification was within mucinous secretions in a case of intermediate-grade micropapillary DCIS.

such as comedo sub-type, large cell size and nuclear pleomorphism. There has also been an association demonstrated between c-erbB-2 expression and cellular proliferation[12]. C-erbB-2 expression has been shown to correlate strongly with the presence of necrosis.

It is therefore not surprising that the correlations of c-erbB-2 expression and the radiological features of DCIS are similar to those seen between the presence of necrosis and the radiological features of DCIS. C-erbB-2-positive DCIS more commonly

45

2

demonstrates calcification (92% versus 72%), a ductal distribution of calcification (78% versus 57%), rod-shaped calcification (82% versus 54%) and granular calcification (97% versus 86%). C-erbB-2-negative DCIS more commonly displays abnormal mammography without calcification (28% versus 8%)[13]. It can be seen from the above associations that c-erbB-2-positive DCIS more frequently shows calcification with morphological features characteristic of malignancy.

p53 and MIB1

p53 is a tumour supressor gene, which has been described as the "guardian of the genome". Mutated p53 may be assessed immunohistologically and it has been found to be expressed in about 25% of DCIS cases. p53 expression is associated with large cell size and necrosis. Whilst one might therefore expect correlation to exist between p53 expression and the mammographic features of DCIS, we could not find any such relationship[14]. Similarly, MIB1, which is a measure of cellular proliferation and is a nuclear protein expressed by cells not in the G0 (resting phase) of the cell cycle, has not been shown to have statistically significant correlations with the mammographic features of DCIS[14]. This is presumably because MIB1 activity correlates strongly with cellular proliferation but less strongly with necrosis and it is necrosis that is the major determinate of radiological features of DCIS.

Oestrogen and progesterone receptors

Up to 60% of DCIS cases are oestrogen receptor-positive. Oestrogen receptor positivity is found more frequently in DCIS with small cell size and in DCIS which does not contain necrosis. Oestrogen receptors are of particular interest due to the investigation of the role of tamoxifen in preventing local recurrence after wide local excision of DCIS. The more characteristic calcification morphological features of DCIS such as granular and rod-

shaped calcifications are seen more frequently in oestrogen receptor-negative DCIS than in oestrogen receptor-positive cases. Similarly, a ductal distribution of calcification, rod shapes and branching calcifications are seen more frequently in progesterone receptor-negative cases[14].

Diagnosing recurrent DCIS

Postconservation surveillance mammography is especially important in women who have had DCIS treated by wide local excision. Mammography is important for two reasons within this group:

1. At least 50% of women with recurrent DCIS have invasive disease recurrence. Detection before metastasis has occurred is therefore of vital importance.
2. Mammography is the sole method of detecting recurrent DCIS in the vast majority of cases.

A recent study of the mammographic features of locally recurrent DCIS demonstrated 85% of local recurrences were detected solely by mammography and that 95% of recurrent DCIS was visible mammographically[15]. The mammographic feature of locally recurrent DCIS was calcification in 90% of cases. This occurred in the same quadrant as the originally diagnosed disease in 90%. This study also showed that the calcification morphology of recurrent DCIS was the same as that of the original lesion in 82% of cases. Other studies have previously demonstrated that locally recurrent invasive breast cancer also has a tendency to recur with the radiological features of the original tumour. One such study showed that in five out of six patients where the original tumour appeared as microcalcification, the recurrence was also detected due to the presence of microcalcification[16]. It is self-evident from these findings that having the diagnostic mammograms available for comparison will aid the reporting of follow-up mammography in women who have had wide local excision of DCIS.

Unfortunately, calcification is a common finding in the irradiated breast and, in some series, as many as 25% of patients who have had wide local excision followed by radiotherapy develop benign-appearing calcifications. Although with time these calcifications appear coarse and curvilinear in nature, when they first appear they can be faint and pleomorphic and often raise a suspicion of recurrent carcinoma. Calcifications that occur soon after wide local excision with radiotherapy (within the first 18 months) are less likely to be malignant than those that occur at a later time interval[17].

What is the value of detecting DCIS at mammographic screening?

The introduction of mammographic screening has led to a dramatic increase in the number of cases of pure DCIS diagnosed. Twenty to 25% of screen-detected breast cancers are DCIS compared with 5% of symptomatic breast cancer[18,19]. Screening women under 50 years of age is associated with even higher proportions of pure DCIS lesions than those seen when screening women over 50[20].

Ductal carcinoma in situ represents a spectrum of disease. Low grade DCIS has only a 25–50% chance of developing into (low-grade) invasive cancer at 30 years and has low rates of local recurrence when treated by wide local excision[21]. Conversely, high grade DCIS, which is often associated with necrosis, in one small series had a 75% risk of invasive disease with a mean time to recurrence of only 4 years[22]. A more recent study has shown that DCIS with poorly differentiated cytonuclear morphology has a significantly higher risk for the development of invasive carcinoma than DCIS with well differentiated cytonuclear appearance[23].

High grade DCIS is also associated with high grade invasive cancer. High grade invasive cancer carries a poor prognosis unless detected when less than 10 mm in size. DCIS that is of high histological grade and, the presence of necrosis are also known to predict for higher rates of recurrence after treatment by wide local excision[24–27]. Approximately 50% of recurrent lesions following wide local excision of DCIS have associated invasive carcinoma and there is a strong association between the grade of the original lesion and the grade of the recurrent invasive carcinoma[28–30].

Critics of breast screening often claim that the high rates of DCIS seen represent over-diagnosis, many being lesions which would never present clinically and threaten the woman's life[31]. This is compounded by the fact that such lesions may be extensive and therefore frequently require mastectomy to obtain adequate excision. Such criticism would only be valid if screen-detected DCIS lesions were predominantly of low histological grade.

Early studies have compared the histological features of screen-detected and symptomatic DCIS but have used DCIS classifications based on the previously utilised system of distinguishing sub-types based on architectural pattern. These studies found that comedo DCIS was commoner in screen-detected lesions than in lesions presenting symptomatically[32,33]. Since these studies were published, a number of new DCIS classifications have been proposed based on cytological features and/or the presence of necrosis[7,24,34,35]. We have found that DCIS detected by mammographic screening is predominantly of high nuclear grade and only 13% is of low grade. Screen-detected DCIS is also more likely to contain areas of necrosis than symptomatic lesions. The most likely explanation for these findings is suggested by a comparison of the radiological findings of different DCIS sub-types. High grade DCIS more frequently shows abnormal mammographic features than low grade DCIS, which is often mammographically occult. The mammographic calcification found in high grade DCIS and DCIS with necrosis is more characteristic of malignancy, often showing rod and branch shapes. The granular/punctate calcifications seen in low grade DCIS are non-specific and are more likely to be confused with benign processes and possibly not recalled at mammographic screening.

Thus screen-detected DCIS is predominantly of high histological grade. The detection of high grade DCIS by screening is likely to prevent the development of poor prognosis, high grade invasive cancer within a few years and could be important in producing part of the mortality reduction seen in randomised trials of mammographic screening. The sub-type profile of screen-detected DCIS suggests that most lesions would progress to high grade invasive disease within 5–10 years. Preventing such high grade invasive disease is likely to have a significant impact on breast cancer mortality. The small proportion of low grade, non-necrotic DCIS lesions found at mammographic screening indicates that diagnosis of the more indolent forms of DCIS is not common.

We therefore advocate the aggressive investigation of suspicious microcalcification seen at mammographic screening. This should lead to the detection of predominantly high grade DCIS and also enables the diagnosis of otherwise occult co-existing, small, grade 3 invasive carcinomas, which have already arisen within the DCIS lesions. The increased availability of stereotactic core biopsy with digital imaging should mean that an aggressive approach to mammographic calcification should not give rise to high rates of surgical benign biopsy.

Atypical ductal hyperplasia

ADH is a rare condition being seen in only 4% of symptomatic benign biopsies. The incidence increases in association with screen-detected benign microcalcifications (31%) and ADH is seen most commonly as an incidental finding in association with another lesion which has prompted biopsy (in up to 62% of cases[36]). The ability of mammography to detect microcalcification and the use in screening programmes has thus resulted in an increase in the detection of ADH, although some groups have also reported that proliferative diseases of the breast are increasing in prevalence[37]. The significance of the diagnosis lies in the associated increased risk of invasive breast carcinoma which is about four to five times that of the general population[38]. The risk is further increased if the patient has a first-degree relative with breast cancer to 10 times that of the female population[38].

There is wide recognition of the imperfections in the criteria used to diagnose ADH. The original definition of ADH[38] was that of a lesion not showing all the features of DCIS. This has been updated and, although the diagnosis still rests on an absence of all the features of DCIS, additional supporting criteria have been described[7]. Page's view that ADH should be recognised if the cellular changes of DCIS are present but occupy less than two separate duct spaces is widely accepted in the UK[38], although other pathologists recommend that the overall size of the lesion is more important and that a cut-off of 2 mm should be utilised[39]. These criteria recognise essentially the same lesions and there is widespread agreement that ADH is small and focal, measuring less than 2–3 mm in size (Fig. 2.16). It is clear that if such a proliferation is at the edge of a biopsy it may represent the periphery of a more established in situ process and excision of the adjacent tissue should be performed. Similarly, if the appearances

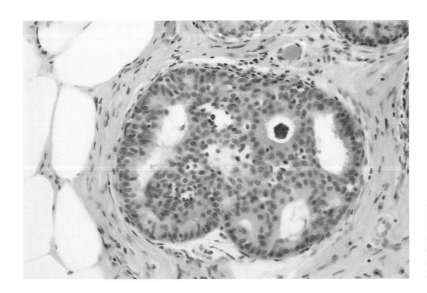

Fig. 2.16
Histological image of an intraductal small-cell epithelial proliferation lacking in the diagnostic features of DCIS. Calcification is noted. The appearances are those of ADH.

equivalent to ADH are seen in a core biopsy, it is not possible for the histopathologist to distinguish ADH from a more established, larger area which would be classified as DCIS.

Thus ADH has, by definition, morphological similarities to low grade DCIS and these entities are also alike in molecular phenotype and DNA characteristics and are jointly different from high-grade DCIS; 36% of ADH and 38% of cribriform DCIS show DNA aneuploidy compared to 93% of morphologically high grade DCIS[40]. A proportion of cases of ADH also fulfil one of the accepted criteria for a neoplasm, being monoclonal in nature[41]. The atypical ductal proliferations of the breast epithelium are thus widely believed to form a spectrum of disease from high grade DCIS at one end to low grade in situ disease and ADH at the other. At the low grade end of this spectrum, ADH and low grade DCIS share common histological and radiological features.

References

1. Evans A, Pinder S, Wilson R et al. Ductal carcinoma in situ of the breast: correlation between mammographic and pathologic findings. Am J Roentgenol 1994; 162: 1307–11.
2. Ceccherini A, Evans AJ, Pinder SE, Wilson ARM, Ellis IO, Yeoman LJ. Is ipsilateral mammography worthwhile in Paget's disease of the breast? Clin Radiol 1996; 51: 35–8.
3. Evans AJ, Wilson ARM, Pinder SE, Ellis IO, Sibbering DM, Yeoman LJ. Ductal carcinoma in situ: imaging, pathology and treatment. Imaging 1994; 6: 171–84.
4. Evans AJ, Wilson ARM, Burrell HC, Ellis IO, Pinder SE. Mammographic features of ductal carcinoma in situ (DCIS) present on previous mammography. Clin Radiol 1999; 54: 644–9.
5. Thomson JZ, Evans AJ, Pinder SE, Burrell HC, Wilson ARM, Ellis IO. Growth pattern of ductal carcinoma in situ (DCIS): a retrospective analysis based on mammographic findings. Br J Cancer 2001; 85: 225–227.
6. Stomper P, Connolly J. Ductal carcinoma in situ of the breast: correlation between mammographic calcification and tumour sub-type. Am J Roentgenol 1992; 159: 483–5.
7. National Coordinating Group for Breast Screening Pathology. Pathology Reporting in Breast Screening Pathology, 2nd ed: NHSBSP Publications no 3, 1997.
8. Silverstein MJ, Poller DN, Waisman JR et al. Prognostic classification of breast ductal carcinoma in situ. Lancet 1995; 345: 1154–7.
9. Holland R, Hendriks JHCL, Vebeek ALM et al. Extent, distribution, and mammographic/histological correlations of breast ductal carcinoma in situ. Lancet 1990; 335: 519–22.

2

10. Holland R, Hendricks J. Microcalcifications associated with ductal carcinoma in situ: mammographic–pathologic correlation. Semin Diagn Pathol 1994; 11: 181–92.

11. Ramachandra S, Machin L, Ashley S et al. Immunohistochemical distribution of c-erbB-2 in in situ breast carcinoma – a detailed morphological analysis. J Pathol 1990; 161: 7–14.

12. Barnes DM, Meyer JS, Gonzalez JG et al. Relationship between c-erbB-2 immunoreactivity and thymidine labelling index in breast carcinoma in situ. Breast Cancer Res Treat 1991; 18: 11–17.

13. Evans AJ, Pinder SE, Ellis IO et al. Correlations between the mammographic features of ductal carcinoma in situ (DCIS) and c-erbB-2 oncogene expression. Nottingham Breast Team. Clin Radiol 1994; 49: 559–62.

14. Evans AJ. Mammographic and pathologic correlations. In: Silverstein, MJ, editor. Ductal Carcinoma in Situ of the Breast. Baltimore: Williams and Wilkins, 1997, pp. 119–24.

15. Liberman L, Van Zee KJ, Dershaw DD, Morris EA, Abramson AF, Samli B. Mammographic features of local recurrence in women who have undergone breast-conserving therapy for ductal carcinoma in situ. Am J Roentgenol 1997; 168: 489–93.

16. Burrell HC, Sibbering DM, Evans AJ. Do mammographic features of locally recurrent breast cancer mimic those of the original tumour? Breast 1996; 5: 233–6.

17. Dershaw DD, Giess CS, McCormick B et al. Patterns of mammographically detected calcifications after breast-conserving therapy associated with tumor recurrence. Cancer 1997; 79: 1355–61.

18. Andersson I, Aspegren K, Janzon L et al. Mammographic screening and mortality from breast cancer: the Malmo mammographic screening trial. Br Med J 1988; 297: 943–8.

19. Smart C, Myers M, Gloecker L. Implications from SEER data on breast cancer management. Cancer 1978; 41: 787–9.

20. Evans WP, Starr AL, Bennos ES. Comparison of the relative incidence of impalpable invasive breast carcinoma and ductal carcinoma in situ in cancers detected in patients older and younger than 50 years of age. Radiology 1997; 204: 489–91.

21. Page DL, Dupont WD, Rogers LW, Jensen RA, Schuyler PA. Continued local recurrence of carcinoma 15–25 years after a diagnosis of low-grade ductal carcinoma in situ of the breast treated only by biopsy. Cancer 1995; 76: 1197–200.

22. Dean L, Geshchicter CF. Conedocarcinoma of the breast. Arch Surg 1938; 36: 225–34.

23. Eusebi V, Feudale E, Foschini MP et al. Long-term follow-up of in situ carcinoma of the breast. Semin Diag Pathol 1994; 11: 223–35.

24. Silverstein MJ, Poller DN, Waisman JR et al. Prognostic classification of breast ductal carcinoma in situ. Lancet 1995; 345: 1154–7.

25. Silverstein MJ, Lagios MD, Craig PH et al. A prognostic index for ductal carcinoma in situ of the breast. Cancer 1996; 77: 2267–74.

26. Fisher ER, Dignam J, Tan-Chiu E et al. Pathological findings from the National Surgical Adjuvant Breast Project (NSABP) eight-year update of protocol B-17. Cancer 1999; 86: 429–38.

27. Solin LJ, I-Tien Y, Kurtz J. Ductal carcinoma in situ (intraductal carcinoma) of the breast treated with breast conserving surgery and definitive irradiation. Cancer 1993; 71: 2532–42.

28. Douglas-Jones AG, Gupta SK, Attanoos RL et al. A critical appraisal of six modern classifications of ductal carcinoma in situ of the breast (DCIS): correlation with grade of associated invasive carcinoma. Histopathology 1996; 29: 397–409.

29. Cadman B, Ostrowski J, Quinn C. Invasive ductal carcinoma accompanied by ductal carcinoma in situ (DCIS): comparison of DCIS grade with grade of invasive component. Breast 1997; 6: 132–7.

30. Lampejo OT, Barnes DM, Smith P, Millis RR. Evaluation of infiltrating ductal carcinoma with a DCIS component: correlation of the histologic type of the in situ component with grade of the infiltrating component. Semin Diag Pathol 1994; 11: 215–22.

31. Baum M. Review of ABC of breast disease. J Med Screening 1995; 2: 233–4.

32. Evans AJ, Pinder SE, Ellis IO et al. Screening detected and symptomatic ductal carcinoma in situ. Mammographic features with pathologic correlation. Radiology 1994; 191: 237–40.

33. Bellamy CO, McDonald C, Salter DM et al. Non-invasive ductal carcinoma of the breast: the relevance of histologic categorization. Hum Pathol 1993; 24: 16–23.

34. Poller DN, Silverstein MJ, Galea M et al. Ductal carcinoma in situ of the breast. A proposal for a new simplified histological classification. Association between cellular proliferation and c-erbB-2 protein expression. Mod Pathol 1994; 7: 257–62.

35. Holland R, Peterse JL, Millis RR et al. Ductal carcinoma in situ: a proposal for a new classification. Semin Diagn Pathol 1994; 11: 167–80.

36. Stomper PC, Cholewinski SP, Penetrante RB, Harlos JP, Tsangaris TN. Atypical hyperplasia: frequency and mammographic and pathologic relationships in excisional biopsies guided with mammography and clinical examination. Radiology 1993; 189: 667–71.

37. Schnitt SJ, Jimi A, Kojiro M. The increasing prevalence of benign proliferative breast lesions in Japanese women. Cancer 1993; 71: 2528–31.

38. Page DL, Dupont WD, Rogers LW, Rados MS. Atypical hyperplastic lesions of the female breast. A

long-term follow-up study. Cancer 1985; 55:
2698–708.

39. Tavassoli FA, Norris HJ. A comparison of the results
of long-term follow-up for atypical intraductal
hyperplasia and intraductal hyperplasia of the
breast. Cancer 1990; 65: 518–29.

40. Crissman JD, Visscher DW, Kubus J. Image
cytophotometric DNA analysis of atypical

hyperplasias and intraductal carcinomas of the
breast. Arch Pathol Lab Med 1990; 114: 1249–53.

41. Lakhani SR, Collins N, Stratton MR, Sloane JP.
Atypical ductal hyperplasia of the breast: clonal
proliferation with loss of heterozygosity on
chromosomes 16q and 17p. J Clin Pathol 1995; 48:
611–15.

Chapter

3

Invasive carcinoma

Andy Evans and Sarah Pinder

Introduction

Calcification is a common mammographic feature of invasive carcinoma. In particular, in a recent series from Milan, Italy, the percentage of non-palpable invasive cancers displaying calcifications was shown to correlate strongly with age. In this series, calcification was seen mammographically in 88% of the invasive cancers detected under the age of 40 but only 22% of similar tumours in women over the age of 70[1]. One of the reasons for this trend was that an extensive intraductal component was much more frequently found in younger women; an EIC was found in 36% of women aged under 40 but this dropped to 6.5% in women aged over 70 (see Table 3.1). This study also showed that associated DCIS not to the extent of representing extensive intraductal component, was also commoner in younger women (see Table 3.2).

The mean invasive size of screen-detected carcinomas associated with both comedo and non-comedo suspicious calcifications in Nottingham is 14 mm[2]. The only mammographic sign associated with smaller invasive cancers is architectural distortion. This may be difficult to identify and therefore the recognition of any associated calcification is a useful mammographic feature for the detection of small invasive cancers.

Calcification also has strong correlations with the histological grade of invasive breast cancers. Comedo calcification, in particular, is strongly associated with grade 3 invasive cancer (Figs 3.1 and 3.2). Eighteen and a half per cent of grade 3 invasive cancers display comedo calcification mammographically compared with less than 3% for grade 2 and grade 1 invasive cancers. Similar, but less strong, associations are seen between granular microcalcifications (non-comedo suspicious calcification) and the grade of invasive cancer. In total, 40% of grade 3 invasive cancers show some form of mammographic microcalcification, whereas only 20% or fewer cases of grade 2 and grade 1 invasive cancers display mammographic microcalcification[2] (see Table 3.3). Other studies have confirmed that correlation between invasive tumour grade and calcification[1]. We have, however, been unable to show any association between the presence of mammographic calcification and lymph node stage or vascular invasion status[2].

Why is calcification associated with grade 3 invasive cancers?

High-grade DCIS tends to give rise to high-grade invasive cancer, and low-grade DCIS to low-grade invasive cancer[3–5]. This association between grade of invasive cancer and DCIS grade is present whatever grading system is used. On average, 67% of invasive cancers associated with high-grade DCIS using five different grading systems were histologically grade 3. Using the Van

Table 3.1 Correlations between age and mammographic calcification in invasive breast cancer[1]

Age (years)	No. of cases	Cancers with microcalcifications (%)
>40	33	87.9
40–49	167	68.3
50–59	283	54.4
60–69	156	40.4
≥70	46	21.7

Table 3.2 Distribution of invasive tumour histology (%) according to patient age[1]

	<40 years	40–49 years	50–59 years	60–69 years	≥70 years
Ductal + DCIS (%) but not EIC	18.2	22.2	14.5	12.8	8.7
Ductal + EIC (%)	36.4	17.4	15.5	12.2	6.5

Table 3.3 Correlations between mammographic calcification and the grade of prevalent round screen-detected invasive breast carcinoma[2]

Mammographic feature	Tumour grade		
	Grade 1 *n* (%)	Grade 2 *n* (%)	Grade 3 *n* (%)
Comedo calcification	2 (2.6)	2 (2.4)	5 (18.5)
Non-comedo suspicious calcification	7 (9.0)	10 (12.1)	5 (18.5)
Benign calcifications	13 (16.7)	17 (20.5)	11 (40.7)

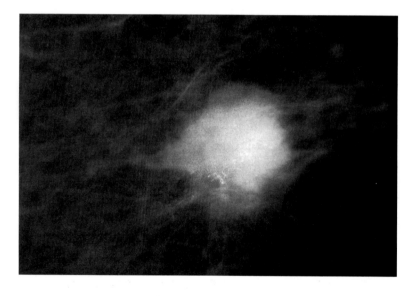

Fig. 3.1
Mammographic image showing an ill-defined mass with associated suspicious microcalcification. Histologically, this represented a grade 3 invasive carcinoma.

Nuys system as many as 75% of invasive cancers associated with high-grade DCIS are grade 3.

The vast majority (>90%) of high-grade DCIS cases display mammographic calcification, which is often of comedo morphology. Low-grade DCIS only display mammo-graphic calcification in 50–60% of cases[6,7]. As few cases of low-grade DCIS are necrotic, the majority of the calcifications are granular or punctate. These findings explain the association between calcification, particularly calcification of comedo type and the grade of associated invasive cancer.

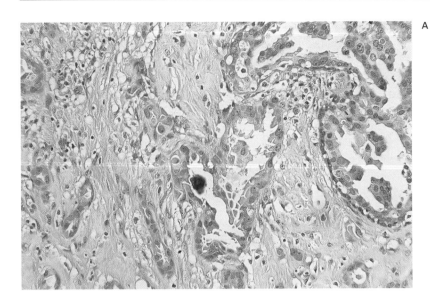

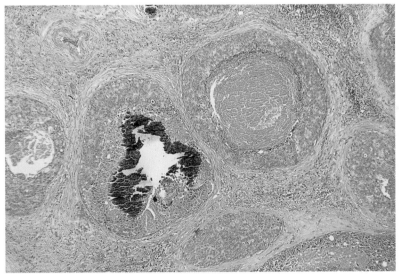

Fig. 3.2
(A) Calcification in the invasive component of a grade 2/3 carcinoma. (B) Calcification in high-grade DCIS in the centre of a grade 3 invasive carcinoma.

The grade of DCIS associated with invasive cancers has been shown to correlate with both disease-free interval and survival. These data indicate the biological importance of DCIS and that the grade of associated DCIS has biological significance. The strong associations that exist between the grade of invasive cancers and the grade of DCIS from which they arose may, at least in part, explain the above associations.

The importance of DCIS in enabling the detection of small grade 3 invasive tumours

Data from the Swedish two-counties study has shown that grade 3 invasive cancers less than 10 mm in size have an excellent prognosis[8]. This compares markedly with the poor prognosis of large grade 3 invasive cancers. In a recent study looking at screen-detected

3

grade 3 invasive cancers, we found that 54% had DCIS surrounding the invasive tumours (Fig. 3.3). Twenty-one per cent had no associated DCIS and 25% had DCIS which was confined to within the invasive component (minimal DCIS)[9].

As can be seen from Table 3.4, the presence of surrounding DCIS in histological grade 3 screen-detected invasive cancer is associated with smaller size of the invasive component compared with similar invasive cancers with either no DCIS or minimal DCIS. It can also be seen that there is a non-significant trend to node negativity in histological grade 3 invasive cancers with surrounding DCIS compared with the other two sub-groups[9].

Table 3.5 shows the correlations between the mammographic appearances of screen-detected histological grade 3 invasive cancer and histological size and nodal status.

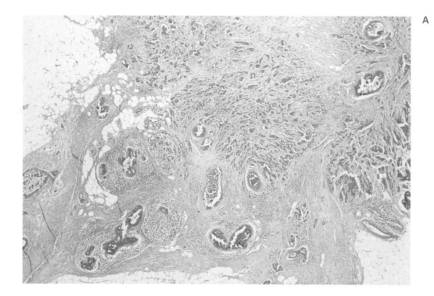

A

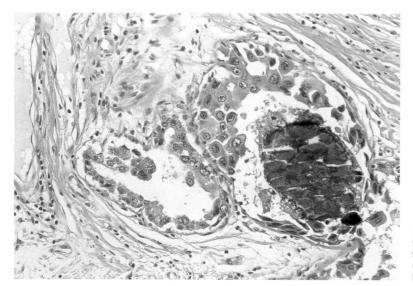

B

Fig. 3.3
(A) Histological image showing a small grade 3 invasive carcinoma (B) associated with surrounding high-grade DCIS.

Table 3.4 Histological size and nodal status of grade 3 tumours by associated DCIS[9]

DCIS status	No. of grade 3 tumours (%)	Size range (mm)	Median size (mm)	Mean size (mm)	No. of grade 3 tumours < 10 mm (%)	Nodal stage		
						Stage 1	Stage 2 or 3	(%)
No DCIS	13	13–35	20	20	0	7	5	(42)[a]
Minimal DCIS	15 (25)	10–30	21	20	2 (13)	8	6	(43)
Surrounding DCIS	33 (54)	1.5–33	14	15	10 (30)	23	7	(28)

[a]Numbers in parentheses are percentages

3

Table 3.5 Histological size and nodal status of grade 3 tumours according to mammographic appearance[9]

Mammographic appearance	No. of grade 3 tumours (%)	Size range (mm)	Median size (mm)	Mean size (mm)	No. of grade 3 tumours < 10 mm (%)	Nodal stage			
						Stage 1	Stage 2	Stage 3	Stage 2 or 3
Granular/punctate calcification	11 (18)	6–28	19	16	2 (18)	6	5	2	5 (43)
Comedo calcification	14 (23)	1.5–33	12	15	6 (43)	10	3	1	4 (29)
All suspicious calcification	25 (42)	1.5–33	19	15	8 (32)	16	8	1	9 (36)
Calcification no mass	6 (10)	1.5–28	13	13	2 (33)	5	1	0	1 (17)
Calcification with mass	19 (32)	6–33	19	19	5 (26)	11	7	1	8 (42)
Mass without calcification	35 (58)	5–35	18	18	4 (11)	22	7	4	11 (33)

It can be seen from Table 3.5 that calcific tumours were more likely to be less than or equal to 10 mm in size than non-calcific tumours (32% versus 11%, $P < 0.05$) (Figs 3.4 and 3.5). This is predominantly because of the high frequency of tumours less than or equal to 10 mm in size in the comedo calcification group. This group represents only 23% of all the tumours but contained 50% of all small tumours. Forty-three per cent of tumours showing comedo calcification were less than or equal to 10 mm in size compared with only 13% of those tumours without this feature[9]. This study indicates that surrounding DCIS is common in histological grade 3 screen-detected cancers and this enables detection mammographically at a smaller size than grade 3 tumours without surrounding DCIS. It is therefore self-evident that detection and aggressive investigation of mammographic calcification is an important part of any mammographic screening programme.

Extensive in situ component

The prognostic importance of an extensive in situ component (EIC) is controversial. Although it has been found that invasive cancers with an EIC have fewer nodal

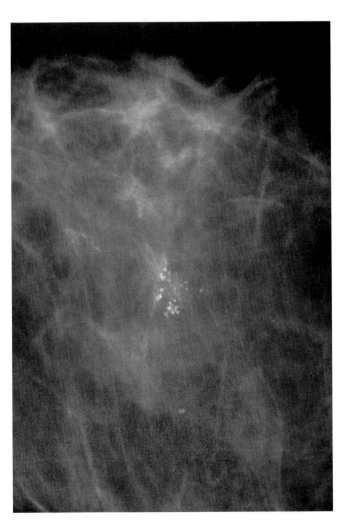

Fig. 3.4
Mammographic image showing a small cluster of pleomorphic calcification. Histology demonstrated high-grade DCIS with a 4-mm invasive grade 3 carcinoma.

3

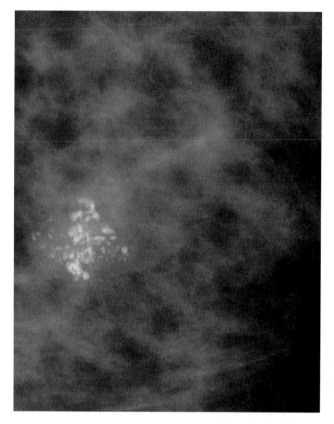

Fig. 3.5
Mammographic image showing a coarse cluster of pleomorphic calcifications with no obvious associated mammographic mass. Histological examination showed an area of high-grade DCIS with an associated grade 3 ductal carcinoma of no specific type.

metastases and a significantly better 10-year survival, tumours with EIC were also of lower histological grade[10]. It may well be that the presence of an EIC is not an independent prognostic factor when histological grade and type are taken into account. This question would best be resolved in a large series including multivariate analysis. The presence of an EIC is practically at this time of greater importance in patients being considered for breast-conserving surgery. At a meeting of the European Organisation for Research into the Treatment of Cancer (EORTC) it was concluded that the principle risk factor for breast relapse after breast-conserving treatment was a large residual burden and the main source of this burden was EIC[11]. The presence of EIC may not be clinically

apparent and one of the important roles of preoperative mammography in patients being considered for breast-conserving therapy is to demonstrate mammographically the presence of an EIC (Figs 3.6 and 3.7).

Predicting invasion in mammographically detected microcalcification

It is important to attempt to diagnose preoperatively invasive disease associated with DCIS. This allows the patient to undergo a single therapeutic operation with appropriate staging/treatment of the axilla. Because axillary metastases are extremely rare in patients with pure DCIS, routine axillary

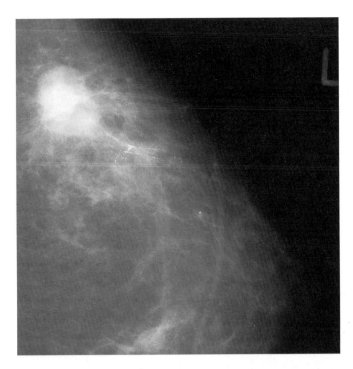

Fig. 3.6
An ill-defined mass representing an invasive carcinoma with extensive associated high-grade DCIS growing towards the nipple. The extent of the DCIS made this lesion unsuitable for breast-conserving surgery.

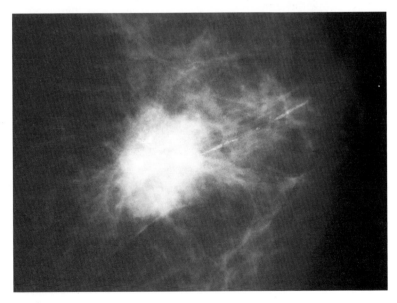

Fig. 3.7
Mammographic image showing an ill-defined mass which represented an invasive carcinoma with obvious ductal calcification extending towards the nipple.

lymph node dissection is inappropriate in such patients. However, multiple studies have shown that about 20% of patients with pure DCIS diagnosed on core biopsy in fact have an invasive focus on surgical excision.

Lagios et al., in a paper from the 1980s, suggested that occult invasion was negligible in association with mammographic clusters below 25 mm in size but showed a 44% risk of invasion in clusters larger than 25 mm[12].

Table 3.6 Calcium cluster size and risk of invasion[13]

Cluster size (mm)	DCIS (*n*)	Invasive
< 11	22	5 (18%)
11–30	24	13 (35%)
31–60	22	10 (31%)
> 60	13	7 (35%) $P = 0.49$

This has not been our personal experience with screen-detected DCIS as we have found a number of invasive foci in small calcification clusters. This prompted us to look in more detail at predicting invasive foci within calcification clusters. In a recent study[13], we looked at 116 patients presenting with malignant mammographic calcification, without an associated mammographic or palpable mass. The final diagnosis was DCIS in 78 patients and DCIS plus an invasive focus in 38 cases (33%). In women where core biopsy made a malignant diagnosis, the sensitivity for invasion was 55% and the negative predictive value of core biopsy for invasion was 79%. We have found that invasive foci were equally common in patients with comedo or granular-type calcification. However, in the five patients with punctate calcification, we did not find any invasive foci.

Table 3.6 shows the relationship between calcification cluster size and risk of invasion; it can be seen that there is not a significant correlation between cluster size and risk of invasion. The mean size of pure DCIS clusters was 32 mm and the mean size of DCIS clusters with an invasive focus was not significantly different (35 mm). We have, however, found a significant trend between increasing number of calcific flecks and the risk of invasive disease (Table 3.7). The risk of invasion in clusters comprising fewer than 10 flecks, 10–40 flecks and over 40 flecks of calcification was 15%, 24% and 43%, respectively ($P < 0.05$).

There was a significant correlation between the DCIS grade predicted on core biopsy and the surgical DCIS grade. We also found that there was a correlation between the DCIS core grade and the risk of invasion. If high-grade DCIS was found on core biopsy, there was a 37% risk of invasive disease, whereas none of the cases with intermediate- or low-grade DCIS on core biopsy had an invasive focus at surgical excision.

Combining these features was found significantly to predict for invasion; we found a 48% risk of invasion in those cases with high-grade DCIS diagnosed on core biopsy and more than 40 calcifications. Conversely, there was only a 15% risk of invasion in clusters diagnosed preoperatively as high-grade DCIS containing fewer than 40 flecks (see Table 3.8).

It is interesting to speculate as to why the number of calcifications is a better predictor of an invasive focus than the mammographic

Table 3.7 Number of cluster calcifications and risk of invasion[13]

Number	DCIS (n)	Invasive
1–10	11	2 (15%)
11–40	45	14 (24%)
> 40	25	19 (43%) $P < 0.05$

Table 3.8 Core DCIS grade and cluster calcification number – prediction of risk of invasion[13]

	High grade		Intermediate or low grade	
Number	DCIS	Invasive	DCIS	Invasive
< 40	27	4 (15%)	11	0
< 40	11	10 (48%)	5	0
Total	38	14	16	0

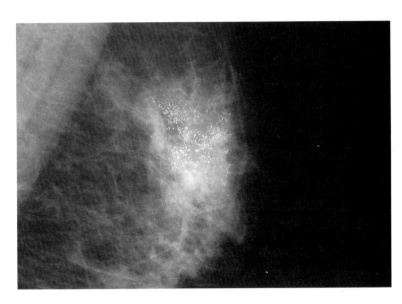

Fig. 3.8
Mammographic image showing an extensive area of DCIS with over 40 calcific flecks demonstrated. Such a case with the presence of a core biopsy showing high-grade DCIS has an almost 50% chance of an invasive focus. Given this fact, a lymph node sample or sentinel node biopsy may be indicated in these circumstances.

cluster size. A possible explanation is that the number of calcifications is a more accurate predictor of the total amount of breast tissue involved by DCIS. A focus of DCIS 60 mm in maximum extent involving just one duct space where a focus 60 × 60 mm in area will have a much higher total volume of breast tissue involved by DCIS than a 60 mm single duct of DCIS. There will therefore be a higher risk of an invasive focus in the former. The *presence* of calcifications is also likely to be a predictor of high-grade disease and therefore an increased risk of an invasive focus.

We conclude that if patients have high-grade DCIS on core and more than 40 flecks of calcification on their mammogram, the risk of invasion is almost 50% (Fig. 3.8). In this group, an axillary staging procedure such as a lymph node sample or a sentinel node biopsy may be appropriate at the same time as primary excision of the lesion. An alternative management strategy would be to try and diagnose the invasive focus preoperatively by more extensive sampling of the lesion with a vacuum-assisted biopsy.

Is calcification an independent prognostic feature?

A recent paper by Laslo Tabar et al. has suggested that the presence of casting calcification is an independent prognostic feature for invasive screen-detected breast cancer that are less than 15 mm in size[14]. In this paper, 14% of women with 1-mm to 9-mm tumours had casting-type calcification on mammography.

However, this group, surprisingly, accounted for 73% of all breast cancer deaths ($P < 0.001$). In this study, the majority of breast cancer deaths also occurred in women who were lymph node-negative. This paper suggested that histological grade was not a reliable predictor of outcome; this is also an unusual finding in any series of invasive breast carcinoma. At our institution we have been unable to replicate these findings. In a similar study, we found that comedo calcification was not a prognostic factor, even before adjusting for tumour grade. Lymph node status was the most powerful predictor of death in our series of patients. We did, however, confirm that histological grade appears to be a less important prognostic factor in small screen-detected invasive cancers. It is difficult to explain the disparity of the findings between these two studies. It may be that histological sampling of areas of DCIS to look for occult areas of invasion and sampling of lymph nodes for small metastases was less thorough in the 1970s compared to more modern pathological examination.

Is spontaneous resolution of breast calcification a sign of malignancy?

A recent study from Guildford and London has shown that spontaneously resolving breast microcalcification is uncommon, being seen in 0.03% of screening mammograms[15]. This incidence is in keeping with previous studies. This study showed that women with clearly benign resolving microcalcification were not at increased risk of developing invasive breast cancer. However, of the 22 women with indeterminate resolving microcalcification, eight (36%) developed carcinoma. One of these lesions was a radial scar with a focus of lobular carcinoma in situ; the other seven cases were invasive carcinoma predominantly of ductal type. The authors suggest that resolution of indeterminate microcalcification should prompt full investigation and close follow-up.

References

1. Ferranti C, Coopmans de Yoldi G, Biganzoli E et al. Relationship between age, mammographic features and pathological tumour characteristics in non-palpable breast cancer. Br J Radiol 2000; 73: 698–705.
2. De Nunzio MC, Evans AJ, Pinder SE et al. Correlations between the mammographic features of screen-detected invasive breast cancer and pathological prognostic factors. Breast 1996; 5: 1–4.
3. Douglas-Jones AG, Gupta SK, Attomoce RL et al. A critical appraisal of six modern classifications of ductal carcinoma in situ of the breast (DCIS): correlation with grade of associated invasive carcinoma. Histopathology 1996; 29: 397–409.
4. Cadman B, Ostrowski B, Quinn C. Invasive ductal carcinoma accompanied by ductal carcinoma in situ (DCIS): comparison of DCIS grade with grade of invasive component. Breast 1997; 6: 132–7.
5. Lampejo OT, Barnes DM, Smith P, Mills RR et al. Evaluation of infiltrating ductal carcinoma with a DCIS component: correlation of the histologic type of the in situ component with grade of the infiltrating component. Semin Diagn Pathol 1994; 11: 215–22.
6. Holland R, Hendriks JH, Vebeek AL, Mravunac M, Shuurmans Stekhoven JH et al. Extent, distribution and mammographic/histological correlations of breast ductal carcinoma in situ. Lancet 1990; 335: 519–22.
7. Evans A, Pinder SE, Wilson R et al. Ductal carcinoma in situ of the breast: correlation between mammographic and pathologic findings. Am J Roentgenol 1994; 162: 1307–11.
8. Tabar L, Dufy SW, Vitak B. The natural history of breast carcinoma: what have we learned from screening? Cancer 1999; 86: 449–62.
9. Evans AJ, Pinder SE, Snead DR et al. The detection of DCIS at mammographic screening enables the diagnosis of small, grade 3 invasive tumours. Br J Cancer 1997; 75: 542–4.
10. Matsukuma A, Enjoji M, Toyoshima S. Ductal carcinoma of the breast. An analysis of the proportion of intraductal and invasive components. Pathol Res Prac 1991; 187: 62–7.
11. Van Dongen JA, Fentiman IS, Harris JR et al. In situ breast cancer: the EORTC consensus meeting. Lancet 1989; ii: 25–7.
12. Lagios M, Westdahl PR, Margolin FR, Rose MR et al. Ductal carcinoma in situ. Relationship of extent of non-invasive disease to the frequency of occult invasion, multicentricity, lymph node metastases

3

and short-term treatment failures. Cancer 1982; 50: 1309–14.

13. Bagnall MJC, Evans AJ, Wilson ARM et al. Predicting invasion in mammographically detected microcalcification. Clin Radiol 2001; 56: 828–32.

14. Tabar L, Chen HR, Duffy SW et al. A novel method for prediction of long-term outcome of women with T1a, T1b and 10–14-mm invasive breast cancers: a prospective study. Lancet 2000; 355: 429–33.

15. Seymour HR, Cooke J, Given-Wilson RM. The significance of spontaneous resolution of breast calcification. BRJ 1999; 72: 3–8.

3

Chapter

4

Fine-needle aspiration cytology and core biopsy of mammographic microcalcification

Andy Evans and Sarah Pinder

Introduction

Fine-needle aspiration cytology (FNAC) has been used to aid the diagnosis of mammographic microcalcification for many years. A recent review of the literature comparing FNAC with core biopsy has shown that the absolute sensitivity of core biopsy is higher than that of FNAC. This is particularly so if the procedures are performed stereotactically. Stereo FNAC has an absolute sensitivity of 62% compared with stereo core biopsy at 91%. Ultrasound-guided core biopsy is also superior to ultrasound FNAC but the difference is less marked, with the absolute sensitivity of ultrasound FNAC being 83% and that of ultrasound core biopsy 97%[1]. This reduced sensitivity of FNA compared with core seen in the literature is also mirrored by practise in the UK breast screening programme where FNAC has an absolute sensitivity of 54% compared with an absolute sensitivity of 75% for core biopsy[2].

Microcalcifications are particularly difficult to biopsy compared with mass lesions. This is true both for core biopsy and for FNAC. The absolute sensitivity of FNAC when biopsying microcalcification can be high, for example in a particularly good series an absolute sensitivity of 71% was obtained[3]. In general, however, the absolute sensitivity of FNAC is lower and, in particular, in the diagnosis of DCIS is only in the region of 53%[4]. Although the lower absolute sensitivity of FNAC in the diagnosis of DCIS is of concern, the major issue when using FNAC in the diagnosis of microcalcification is the unreliability of FNAC to make a definitive diagnosis of benignity. For example, in a series from Guildford, even though the absolute sensitivity was 71%, 36% of lesions with C1 or C2 cytology were malignant[3]. Similarly, prior to 1994 when core biopsy was introduced in our unit, we found that 28% of calcification cases with a benign cytology were malignant on surgical excision. This is due largely to the fact that FNAC is unable to confirm whether the sample was taken in the right place or whether there was a geographical miss (sampling error). Whilst it is possible to look for microcalcification on FNAC specimens, it is our experience that they are rarely seen. In addition, the resolution of histology/cytology for calcification is much smaller than mammography and even the presence of calcification on a cytology specimen cannot confidently confirm accurate sampling of the lesion. This contrasts with core biopsy specimen radiography, which has been shown in many series to be highly accurate in confirming adequate sampling of the lesion.

Another factor to be taken into account when deciding whether to perform FNAC or core biopsy on an area of microcalcification is patient comfort. A recent study from London UK, asked patients to rate the procedure pain on a fixed-interval rating scale. This showed that there was no difference in the pain produced by core biopsy, FNAC or cyst aspiration. This study found a weak negative correlation between pain and the amount of local anaesthetic used[5]. Patient comfort is therefore not a reason to use FNAC rather than core biopsy.

Concern has been expressed regarding malignant cell displacement at core biopsy. This may, however, be seen also with FNAC[6,7]. Malignant cell displacement does occur with both procedures, but the cells appear to be non-viable; there is a very strong relationship between the frequency of malignant cell displacement and the time between biopsy and surgery. If the biopsy to surgery interval is less than 15 days, tumour displacement is seen in 42% of cases. This frequency reduces to 15% at > 28 days[8]. In Steve Parker's large multicentre study, tumour track recurrence was not seen in almost 1000 cancers diagnosed by core biopsy[9].

Core biopsy

The widespread introduction of automated guns for image-guided core biopsy in the mid 1990s was a significant advance in non-operative diagnosis of mammographic microcalcification. Stereotactically-guided core biopsy of indeterminate calcification allows accurate diagnosis of the majority of microcalcification clusters. The ability to perform specimen radiography to confirm the presence of representative calcification within the specimens is a significant advantage over FNA (Fig. 4.1). The more recent widespread use of digital imaging has further enhanced the ability of stereotactic core biopsy to accurately diagnose microcalcification. It has, however, also become clear that there are a number of cases where image-guided core biopsy significantly "understages" malignant microcalcification. The use of more invasive image-guided procedures to address this problem will be dealt with in a separate chapter.

Core biopsy equipment

Studies on the yields obtained with different core biopsy guns show that the Manan gun (Fig. 4.2) and the Bard gun (Fig. 4.3) give particularly good yield of tissues[10]. The use of disposable Temno needles is associated with particularly poor yields. Although when using upright stereotactic devices a 10-cm length needle is usually adequate, in women with a large breast compressed thickness, it is occasionally useful to use a 13-cm length needle. Use of longer needles, such as a 16-cm needle, is often difficult using upright stereotactic equipment because the tube head may be unable to swing into position due to the projection of the gun. In women with a very small breast compressed thickness, difficulties can arise when performing stereotactic core biopsy. To avoid hitting the tabletop, it is necessary to either use a c-arm or to fire the gun from outside the breast.

The use of a short-throw gun is associated with very poor tissue yields and the long-throw (23-mm) gun should be used at all times (Figs 4.4 and 4.5). Fourteen-gauge needles should be used when performing stereotactic core biopsy of microcalcifications as it has been shown that the preoperative diagnosis of malignancy is significantly poorer if smaller gauge needles are used[11]. We have recently investigated the use of 12-gauge needles to diagnose mammographic microcalcifications. We have found that both specimen X-ray positivity and preoperative diagnosis of DCIS and invasive disease was identical when using 14- and 12-gauge needles[12]. We have therefore continued to use 14-gauge needles when performing stereotactic core biopsy of microcalcifications.

Performing stereotactic core biopsy of

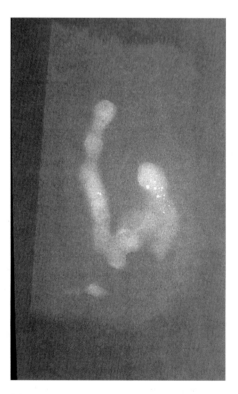

Fig. 4.1
Specimen radiograph showing multiple flecks of calcifications.

4

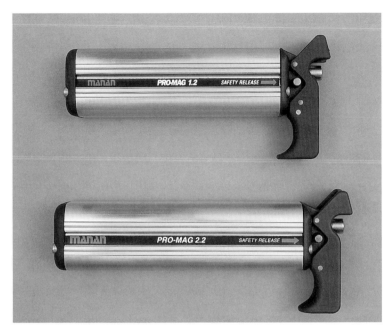

Fig. 4.2
The Manan long- and short-throw guns. We would recommend use of the long-throw gun at all times.

4

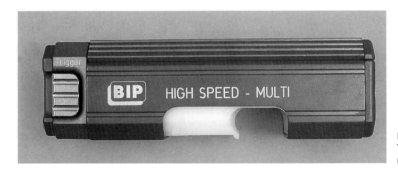

Fig. 4.3
The Bard gun previously manufactured by BIP.

microcalcification is difficult if only film-screen stereotaxis is available. The time lapse between taking a stereo pair and being able to view the image and adjust needle position means that sampling errors are common. In our experience, using film-screen upright stereotaxis, a positive specimen radiograph was only obtained in just over 50% of cases. Indeed, the absolute sensitivities for diagnosing pure DCIS cases using film-screen stereotaxis in our centre was only 34%, although the absolute sensitivity when biopsying microcalcification that contained an invasive focus was slightly higher at 41%. When using film-screen stereotaxis, only two or three check pairs were obtained during the whole procedure. If more stereotactic pairs were taken, the patient was often unable to tolerate the lengthening of the procedure. Complete sensitivities using film-screen stereotaxis were also poor, being 52% for pure DCIS and 59% for DCIS with an invasive focus.

The introduction of digital stereotaxis has enabled the use of many more check pairs during a biopsy procedure. On average, nine check pairs are taken at our institution when performing stereotactic core biopsy. This allows very precise placement of the needle

4

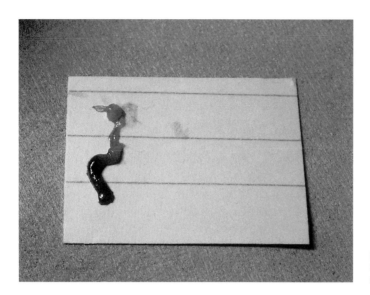

Fig. 4.4
Photograph of a core biopsy performed using the long-throw (23 mm) gun.

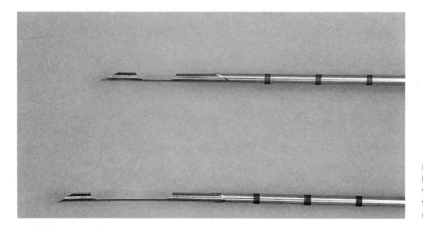

Fig. 4.5
Photograph of short- and long-throw needles. We recommend the use of the long-throw needle at all times.

before firing and also shortens the interval between obtaining an adequate position and firing, thus the patient has less time to move out of position. With the introduction of digital stereotaxis our calcification retrieval rate immediately rose from 55% to 85%. Our absolute sensitivity for the diagnosis of pure DCIS rose from 34% to 69%, and the complete sensitivity from 52% to 94%. This complete sensitivity of 94% indicates that a geographical miss of calcifications using digital equipment is unusual. With the intro-

duction of digital stereotaxis, our absolute sensitivity for diagnosing clusters containing an invasive focus rose from 41% to 67%, and the complete sensitivity from 59% to 86%[13]. Given further experience of the use of digital stereotaxis, our calcification retrieval rate for microcalcific lesions is now 96% and our absolute sensitivity for diagnosing pure DCIS is now 81%. These figures indicate that the results of upright digital stereotaxis (Fig. 4.6) are similar to those achieved with prone table stereotactic biopsies.

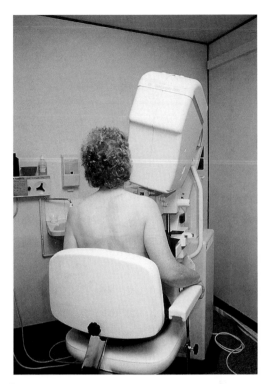

Fig. 4.6
Photograph of a woman undergoing upright stereotactic core biopsy.

The use of the prone table (Fig. 4.7) nevertheless has some advantages over the use of upright digital stereotaxis. Patients in the prone position very rarely faint and patient movement during the procedure is also less common. When performing prone table stereotactic biopsy the skin entry site is also hidden from the patient. This is a particular advantage if blood vessels are incidentally biopsied during the procedure. Conversely, there are disadvantages to the use of the prone table, including the cost of the equipment, the fact that the prone table can only be used for stereotactic biopsies and the large size of the equipment. Radiographic positioning with the prone table is different from radiographic positioning using routine mammographic equipment; positioning skills therefore take some time to acquire. Thus the advantages of upright digital stereo-taxis are that the machine can be used for routine mammography when stereotactic procedures are not being performed, radiographers are used to the positioning skills required to perform the biopsy and that the

4

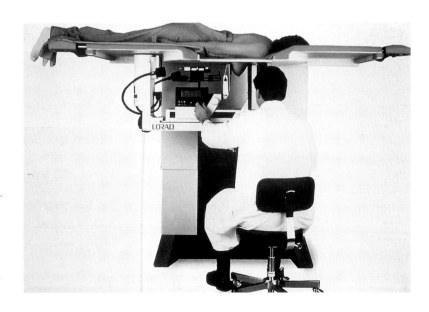

Fig. 4.7
Photograph of a woman undergoing a dedicated prone table biopsy.

cost of a digital add-on is less than the cost of purchasing a dedicated prone table.

Acquiring specimen radiographs promptly is important when performing stereotactic core biopsies of microcalcifications[14]. If immediate specimen radiography is available it means that the number of cores taken can be tailored to the amount of microcalcification present on the specimen radiographs. The use of film-screen specimen radiographs introduces a significant delay between performing the biopsy and knowing how successful the biopsy has been. Therefore the use of digital imaging to provide immediate specimen radiography is very helpful as there is no delay between performing the biopsy and knowing whether the biopsy has been successful or not.

It also means that if the specimen radiograph is negative, further cores can be taken without delay.

Performing stereotactic core biopsy

Before image-guided biopsy is performed it is important that physical examination has been conducted to assess palpability of the lesion. This information is important as it indicates whether wire localisation will be required if the lesion is shown to be malignant. If a physical examination is only performed after the biopsy it is often unclear whether the lesion is palpable or just a postprocedure haematoma (Fig. 4.8A,B). It is also

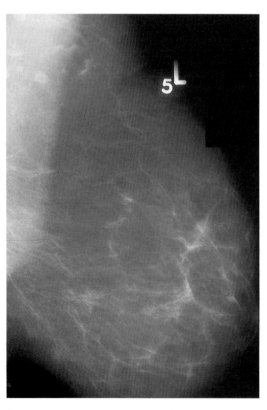

A

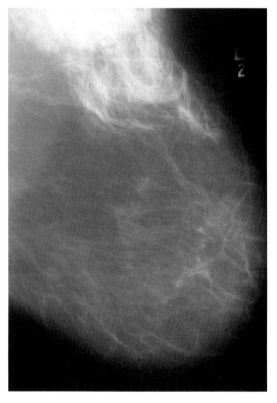

B

Fig. 4.8
Mammogram before and after the freehand core biopsy showing a postprocedural haematoma with diffuse infiltration of the fat in the upper breast.

helpful for the patient to have previously met the member of staff who will give them their biopsy result. The only contraindication to stereotactic core biopsy is anti-coagulation. Before the biopsy is performed it is important to explain to the patient the nature of their abnormality and how core biopsy will help. Whether the patient's consent to the procedure is verbal or written is immaterial. The patient should always be aware before the procedure that repeat biopsies do frequently need to be performed and that core biopsy is not always successful. Before the procedure begins it is of value for the patient to hear the gun being fired as this will help them not to move during the procedure. It is also important to discuss with the radiographer the best plane of approach. The factors important in deciding this are ease of positioning both for the radiographer and the patient, the need for a centimetre or so of normal tissue deep to the lesion and which plane demonstrates the abnormality most clearly. When using upright stereotactic devices, lesions in the upper half of the breast can normally be biopsied in the CC plane. Lesions in the lower medial breast can be biopsied in the mediolateral oblique plane and lesions in the lower outer quadrant are usually biopsied lateral to medial.

Once adequate check images have been produced by the radiographer it is important that the same fleck of calcification is identified on both views. Failure to do this can mean quite large errors in needle positioning. Being able to check the point chosen on the straight scout image can be quite helpful in identifying those cases in which different calcifications have been picked on each check image. The skin is then cleansed and local anaesthetic applied to the skin and down to the lesion, as long as the lesion is not so subtle that it may be obscured by small quantities of air within the local anaesthetic. In such cases, local anaesthetic should only be applied to the skin. The addition of adren-aline is helpful in reducing procedure bleeding. A skin nick is normally performed with an 11-gauge blade. A small hook to move the skin to exactly where the needle tip is quite helpful when performing the procedure. Obtaining optimal needle placement with the use of multiple check images is very worthwhile as the first few cores are often the best. It is our normal practice to perform five cores and then obtain a specimen radiograph. It can be quite frustrating waiting for a specimen radiograph to go through a film processor and we have found the whole procedure of stereotactic core biopsy to be enhanced by the use of digital imaging to provide a specimen image.

The details of how many flecks of calcification are required on a specimen X-ray will be addressed more fully later, but taking five to 10 more cores if required is appropriate. In general, patients much prefer to have their lesion adequately sampled on the first occasion than to come back for a repeat procedure. It has been suggested that if core biopsy specimens are kept in a water-based solution for 3 days, all the calcifications may dissolve. If samples are not going to be fixed and processed promptly, using an ethanol-based solution may prevent calcifications from dissolving[15].

After the procedure, compression should be applied for approximately 5 minutes and the patient is warned against physical exercise for the rest of the day. Patients should also be advised concerning pain control and the possible need for further compression should the wound ooze. Patients should not leave until there has been a clear arrangement made for the patient to receive the result of their biopsy.

How many samples should be taken when biopsying calcification?

A number of studies have looked at the number of core biopsy samples required to make a definitive diagnosis of mammographic microcalcification. A study by Brenner in 1996 compared the diagnostic yield of one to five cores. Not surprisingly, they found a trend towards increasing accuracy with increasing number of cores and that this trend was especially marked in clustered microcalcification[16]. A recent study from London, UK also showed increasing absolute and complete sensitivity with increasing number of cores; six or more cores gave a better diagnostic yield than five cores[17] (see Table 4.1). These results highlight the frequent need to take multiple cores and certainly 10 to 15 cores of microcalcification are not excessive.

A recent study[18] aimed to determine if the number of flecks of calcification retrieved with stereotactic needle core, or the numbers of cores containing calcification, were related to biopsy sensitivity. This paper found that 100% complete sensitivity was obtained once three individual calcific flecks were obtained, but for 100% absolute sensitivity five or more flecks of calcification were required on specimen radiography. This study also showed that for 100% complete sensitivity it was required that two of the cores showed at least one fleck of calcification. For 100% absolute sensitivity, three separate cores each containing at least one fleck were required at specimen radiography. The other important finding of this study was that three specimen X-rays which contained only one or two flecks of calcification gave a benign result, even though the lesion was malignant on excision. The lesson from this study is that if on the initial specimen X-ray only one or two flecks of calcification are obtained further samples should be taken. This will have the dual purpose of helping to exclude malignancy in benign lesions and improve the absolute sensitivity if the lesion is malignant. A sub-analysis within this study showed that the amount of calcification needed to be retrieved at core biopsy was less for clusters containing less than 10 flecks of calcification; the retrieval of two flecks or two cores each containing a fleck gave 100% absolute sensitivity. This finding is likely to be because small calcification clusters are less likely to contain both benign and malignant microcalcifications[18] (see Tables 4.2 and 4.3).

Results of core biopsy of microcalcification

The reported calcification retrieval rate of stereotactic core biopsy is high, in the range of 86% to almost 100%. This high calcification retrieval rate does not, however, lead to a particularly high absolute sensitivity for the

Table 4.1 Relationship between number of cores and sensitivity[17]

Number of cores	2	3	4	5	6+
Microcalcifications: All (*n* = 125)					
Absolute sensitivity	92 (73.6%)	93 (74.4%)	96 (76.8%)	98 (78.4%)	104 (83.2%)
Complete sensitivity	121 (96.8%)	97 (77.6%)	100 (80%)	105 (84%)	108 (86.4%)
Microcalcifications: Indeterminate (*n* = 67)					
Absolute sensitivity	42 (62.7%)	42 (62.7%)	43 (64.2%)	44 (65.7%)	48 (71.6%)
Complete sensitivity	47 (70.1%)	49 (73.1%)	51 (76.1%)	53 (79.1%)	68 (94%)
Microcalcifications: Malignant (*n* = 58)					
Absolute sensitivity	50 (86.2%)	51 (87.9%)	53 (91.4%)	54 (93.1%)	56 (96.6%)
Complete sensitivity	50 (86.2%)	51 (87.9%)	54 (93.1%)	55 (94.8%)	58 (100%)

Table 4.2 Number of calcific elements on specimen radiology versus core histology[18]

Calcifications (n)	Core biopsy result			Sensitivity (%)	
	Normal or benign	Uncertain malignant potential or suspicious	Malignant	Complete	Absolute
0	21	1	3	16	12
1	2	2	7	81.8	63.6
2	1	3	6	90	60
3		1	5	100	83.3
4		2	1	100	33.3
≥ 5			17	100	100
Total	24	9	39		

Table 4.3 Number of cores containing radiographic calcification versus core histology[18]

Calcifications (n)	Core biopsy result			Sensitivity (%)	
	Normal or benign	Uncertain malignant potential or suspicious	Malignant	Complete	Absolute
0	21	1	3	16	12
1	3	6	12	85.7	57.1
2		2	8	100	80
3			8	100	100
4			6	100	100
≥ 5			2	100	100
Total	24	9	39		

diagnosis of malignancy in DCIS lesions and reported absolute sensitivities of stereotactic core biopsy of DCIS lesions are in the order of 44–67%. A non-definitive diagnosis is often due to partial sampling of the lesions. If a low-grade intraductal epithelial proliferation is seen in only two duct spaces, a histological diagnosis of ADH is made; such lesion can only be diagnosed as DCIS if more abnormal ducts are demonstrated. Similarly, if a core biopsy shows part of, or a single, duct space containing a scanty population of more pleomorphic epithelial cells, such as those seen in intermediate- or high-grade DCIS, this is classified as suspicious rather than diagnostic of DCIS. These facts explain why there is a large difference between the calcification retrieval rate and absolute sensitivity for DCIS. Are there particular calcification features which lead to higher or lower sensitivity of core biopsy? Rich et al.[17] demonstrated that in calcifications highly suspicious of malignancy, the absolute sensitivity with six or more core specimens was as high as 97%. However, in the same series, for calcifications graded as a lower risk of malignancy, core biopsy only achieved an absolute sensitivity of 72% with six or more core biopsy samples[17]. Bagnall et al., however, found no difference in the absolute sensitivity of core biopsy when calcifications were classified as either granular or comedo[18]. It is therefore unclear as to whether the absolute sensitivity of core biopsy varies according to radiological appearance of malignant calcification.

How often is malignant calcification "understaged" by core biopsy?

It has been known for some time that a histological diagnosis of ADH may be obtained from a core biopsy of a lesion, which on excision is classified as DCIS. Most series indicate that approximately 50% of lesions with ADH on core show either DCIS or DCIS with invasive cancer at surgical excision[19]. ADH core biopsy results from DCIS lesions are commoner if the mammographic abnormality is a mass rather than microcalcifications. Such underestimation of DCIS lesions by core biopsy and vacuum-assisted biopsy are more common if fewer than 10 cores are taken[20]. Multiple studies have shown that approximately 20% of lesions giving a core biopsy result of DCIS have invasive disease at excision biopsy[21]. Once again, such underestimate of disease is more commonly found if the mammographic abnormality is a mass than in microcalcific cases and underestimation is more common if fewer than 10 cores are taken[20].

Interpreting benign results

Benign core biopsy results from calcific lesions should only be trusted if specimen X-ray shows unequivocal calcification. A benign result from a lesion from which the specimen X-ray only shows one or two flecks of calcification should be interpreted with caution[18]. A repeat biopsy or diagnostic surgical excision should be performed if a histological benign core result is obtained

from a lesion that is highly suspicious of malignancy radiologically. It is also important to note that the presence of calcification on histological examination is no substitute for calcification on the specimen X-ray. The resolution of histology for calcifications is much higher than radiography; thus calcifications can often be found histologically which are incidental and indeed are present in radiologically non-calcific lesions. If no radiographically representative calcification is retrieved and a benign histology result is obtained, the biopsy should either be repeated or the lesion excised. Conversely, if a specimen X-ray shows unequivocal calcification and initial histological examination demonstrates only normal tissue without calcification, further levels into the paraffin-embedded sample should be taken to search for the calcification deeper in the specimen.

References

1. Britton PD. Fine needle aspiration or core biopsy. Breast 1999; 8: 1–4.
2. Britton PD, McCann J. Needle biopsy in the NHS breast screening programme 1996/7: how much and how accurate? Breast 1999; 8: 5–11.
3. Elliott AJ, Cooke JC, McKee G. A 4-year retrospective analysis of screen-detected and stereotactically biopsied microcalcification with emphasis on ways to reduce the number of benign biopsies. Breast 1996; 5: 410–14.
4. Venegas R, Rutgers JL, Cameron VL, Vargas H, Butler JA. Fine-needle aspiration cytology of breast DCIS. Acta Cytol 1994; 38: 16–143.
5. Denton ERE, Ryan S, Beaconfield T, Michell MJ. Image-guided breast biopsy: analysis of pain and discomfort related to technique. Breast 1999; 8: 257–60.
6. Youngson BJ, Cranor M, Rosen PP. Epithelial displacement in surgical breast specimens following needling procedures. Am J Surg Pathol 1994; 18: 896–903.
7. Youngson BJ, Liberman L, Rosen PP. Displacement of carcinomatous epithelium in surgical breast specimens following stereotaxic core biopsy. Am J Clin Pathol 1995; 103: 598–602.
8. Diaz LK, Wiley EL, Venta LA. Are malignant cells displaced by large-gauge needle core biopsy of the breast? Am J Roentgenol 1999; 173: 1303–13.

4

9. Parker SH, Burbank F, Jackman J et al. Percutaneous large-core breast biopsy: a multi-institutional study. Radiology 1994; 3: 359–63.

10. Krebs TL, Berg WE, Severson MJ et al. Large-core biopsy guns: comparison for yield of breast tissue. Radiology 1996; 200: 365–8.

11. Nath ME, Robinson TM, Tobon H, Chough DM, Sumkin JH. Automated large-core needle biopsy of surgically removed breast lesions: comparison of samples obtained with 14-, 16- and 18-guage needles. Radiology 1995; 197: 739–43.

12. Evans AJ, Whitlock JP, Burrell H, et al. A comparison of 14- and 12-gauge needles for core biopsy of suspicious mammographic calcification. Br J Radiol 1999; 72: 1152–4.

13. Whitlock JPL, Evans AJ, Burrell HC et al. Digitally acquired imaging improves upright stereotactic core biopsy of mammographic microcalcifications. Clin Radiol 2000; 55: 374–7.

14. Liberman L, Evans III WP, Dershaw DD et al. Radiography of microcalcifications in stereotaxic mammary core biopsy specimens. Radiology 1994; 190: 223–5.

15. Moritz JD, Luftner-Nagel S, Westerhof JP, J.W. O, Grabbe E. Microcalcifications in breast core biopsy specimens: disappearance at radiography after storage in formaldehyde. Radiology 1996; 200: 361–3.

16. Brenner RJ, Fajardo L, Fisher PR et al. Percutaneous core biopsy of the breast: effect of operator experience and number of samples on diagnostic accuracy. Am J Roentgenol 1996; 166: 341–6.

17. Rich PM, Michell MJ, Humphreys S, Howes GP, Nunnerley HB. Stereotactic 14-G core biopsy of non-palpable breast cancer: what is the relationship between the number of core samples taken and the sensitivity for detection of malignancy? Clin Radiol 1999; 54: 384–9.

18. Bagnall MJC, Evans AJ, Wilson ARM, Burrell HC, Pinder SE, Ellis IO. When have mammographic calcifications been adequately sampled at needle core biopsy? Clin Radiol 2000; 55: 548–53.

19. Liberman L, Cohen MA, Dershaw DD, et al. Atypical ductal hyperplasia diagnosed at stereotaxic core biopsy of breast lesions: an indication for surgical biopsy. Am J Roentgenol 1995; 164: 1111–13.

20. Jackman RJ, Burbank F, Parker SH et al. Stereotactic breast biopsy of non-palpable lesions: determinants of ductal carcinoma in situ underestimation rates. Radiology 2001; 218: 497–502.

21. Liberman L, Dershaw D, Rosen PP et al. Stereotaxic core biopsy of breast carcinoma: accuracy at predicting invasion. Radiology 1995; 194: 379–81.

Large core biopsy for calcification

A. R. M. Wilson

Introduction

The vast majority of microcalcifications can be accurately and effectively sampled using 14-gauge automated core biopsy but, in 10–20% of cases, core biopsy fails to provide a definitive diagnosis[1–4]. The reasons for this include borderline pathological conditions and abnormalities at sites in the breast that are difficult to access using conventional core biopsy[1,2,5,6].

The traditional solution to these sampling problems has been to obtain the tissue required for histological assessment by open surgical biopsy after radiological localisation. However, percutaneous biopsy devices are now available that provide much larger volumes of tissue and these can be used to reduce the need for diagnostic open surgical biopsy for benign conditions and to provide higher rates of preoperative diagnosis for malignant disease[7]. Two different approaches have been developed. One approach is to obtain a single very large core of tissue up to 20 mm in diameter[8,9]. The other approach retrieves multiple contiguous 14-, 11- or 8-French gauge core samples by combining core biopsy with a vacuum system for both acquiring and retrieving tissue samples (vacuum-assisted mammotomy, VAM). VAM is now a routine procedure in many breast diagnostic centres[10,11].

Reasons for failure of conventional core biopsy

Conventional core biopsy obtains separate non-contiguous cores of tissue that are usually sufficient in volume and architectural information to allow for accurate pathological assessment. The most common reason for failure to achieve accurate diagnosis with conventional automated core biopsy is a borderline pathological condition where the pathologist requires a larger volume of tissue than can be obtained by conventional core biopsy to assess the true nature of the pathological process. These include conditions such as radial scar, papillary lesion, mucocele-like lesion, differentiation of low-grade carcinoma in situ from epithelial hyperplasia with atypia (ADH) and the detection of invasive disease associated with in situ carcinoma[12–18]. All of these conditions can calcify and cause diagnostic difficulties for both the radiologist and pathologist.

Another common reason for failure to retrieve any or sufficient representative cellular material from a cluster of microcalcifications is difficulty in accurately targeting the abnormality because of its small size or inaccessible site in the breast. For successful core biopsy, the needle must pass directly through the tissue containing the calcifications at the correct depth. With both upright and prone biopsy devices, successful core biopsy can prove to be difficult or impossible in a proportion of cases because the cluster of calcifications is very small or is at a site difficult to access because of its position in the breast or the habitus of the patient. VAM is ideal in these circumstances as this technique only requires the sampling probe to be placed close to rather than through the area to be sampled. The vacuum and ability to sample tissue in a particular direction means that tissue in an otherwise inaccessible site, for instance at the chest wall and immediately behind the nipple, can be sampled. Using a lateral approach, VAM can also be used to obtain tissue from breasts that are too thin to sample when compressed using the conventional perpendicular approach.

Very large core biopsy

The technique developed by US Surgical Inc. was based on the principle of removing all or most of the abnormality in a single core. This system is called advanced breast biopsy

5

85

instrumentation (ABBI™) and involves the retrieval of a core of tissue from skin to beyond the lesion with a choice 5-, 10- and 20-mm diameter cores. The 20-mm diameter core is the most frequently used. The ABBI™ system is only suitable for use with a prone biopsy table. A variation on the very large core principles similar to ABBI™ is known as SiteSelect™. This device differs in that it is designed to obtain a large core of tissue from the area of the abnormality within the breast without removing the intervening of normal tissue between the skin and the lesion.

The ABBI™ and SiteSelect™ techniques have met with considerable criticism and both are now not used. This is because compared to core biopsy and VAM, the technique is considerably more invasive, more costly, associated with much higher failure and complication rates and is not suitable to be

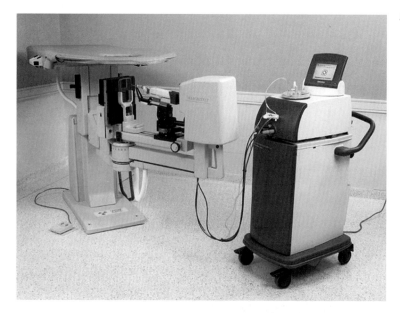

A

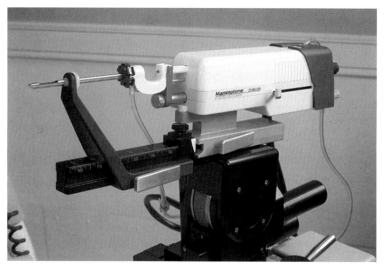

B

Fig. 5.1A&B
The Mammotome ST™ driver and probe shown for use with a prone biopsy table.

5

used in a significant proportion of cases. Although ABBI was initially thought to offer the opportunity to completely excise small lesions, it has not proved to be an acceptable method for treating small malignancies[19]. There are very few cases where either of these very large core techniques offers any advantage over the other less invasive and less costly methods of percutaneous core biopsy.

Vacuum-assisted mammotomy

VAM devices have been developed by US Surgical Inc: Minimally invasive breast biopsy (MIBB™) and Breast Care Ethicon Endosurgery (Mammotome™). The MIBB device could only be used with a prone biopsy table; this device is no longer available. The Mammotome™ has the advantage that it can be used with both prone and upright stereotactic

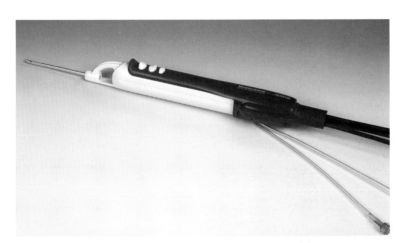

A

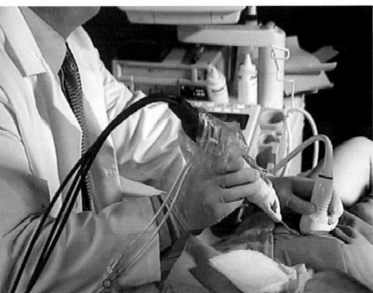

B

Fig. 5.2A&B
The Mammotome HH™ probe used for hand held ultrasound guided biopsy.

devices (Mammotome ST™ – Fig. 5.1) and under ultrasound guidance (Mammotome HH™ – Fig. 5.2)[2,5,20–23]. This device use the principle of a vacuum applied along a double lumen needle to both obtain and retrieve multiple contiguous core samples without the need to remove the needle from the breast for each core specimen[24]. Core size can be 14-, 11- or 8-gauge, delivering specimens of average weight of 35, 100 and 300 mg respectively (Fig. 5.3). This compares to only 17 mg for the average automated 14-gauge core biopsy.

The principles of how the VAM technique works are shown in Fig. 5.4. The Mammotome™ probe consists of three main parts – an outer double lumen probe (1) with a lower section through which suction is applied and an upper sampling chamber, a hollow rotating motorised cutting trocar (2) and an inner specimen retrieval suction trocar (3). The system is computer controlled for ease of use with the sampling sequences pre-programmed by the user. Once placed in the breast, tissue is sucked into the stationary upper sample chamber and the motorised hollow rotating inner cutting trocar separates the specimen. This is then retrieved from the sample site by withdrawing the trocar while applying suction through an inner second trocar. The biopsy probe remains in the breast throughout the sampling process and multiple radial contiguous core samples can be obtained by rotating the whole probe around the biopsy site. Because there is no forward-throw action, sampling of lesions that are small, superficial or close to the chest wall can be easily achieved. VAM is therefore

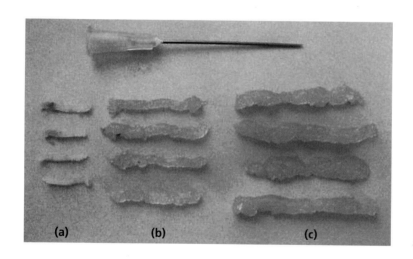

(a) **(b)** **(c)**

Fig. 5.3
Comparison of sample sizes with 14 guage conventional core (a), 11 guage Mammotome (b) and 8 guage Mammotome (c) probes.

1. Stereotactic or ultrasound guidance used to position the probe.

2. Tissue is gently vacuum aspirated into the aperture.

3. The rotating cutter is advanced forward, cutting and capturing a specimen.

4. After the cutter has reached its full forward position, rotation and vacuum cease.

5. The cutter is withdrawn, transporting the specimen to the tissue collection chamber while the outer probe remains in the breast.

Fig. 5.4
Schematic diagrams showing the various stages of the vacuum-assisted mammotomy process.

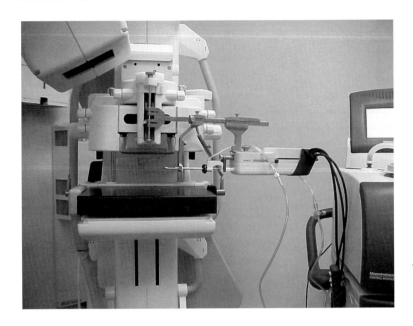

Fig. 5.5
The Mammotome ST™ set up for use with the GE Senovision™ upright digital stereotactic system using the lateral approach.

to be preferred where larger tissue samples are required, when conventional core biopsy has failed to provide a definitive diagnosis, for some very small lesions and for lesions at sites difficult to target with conventional automated core.

VAM is very well tolerated by patients and, despite the needle size, many patients prefer this procedure to automated core biopsy, particularly for stereotactic X-ray-guided biopsy. With automated core biopsy, the noise of the gun firing and the shockwave that this causes in the breast, and the need to remove and reinsert the device for each sample, cause anxiety and distress despite reassurance and prior warning. Anxiety caused by the sampling technique itself is significantly less with the mammotomy technique; there is no loud noise when the sample is obtained and retrieved by the relatively slowly forward and backward rotating cutting inner trocar and the device remains in the breast while multiple specimens are obtained.

VAM retrieves much larger volumes of tis-sue using a rotating cutting trocar and for this reason it is important and necessary to use more local anaesthesia than is usually needed for automated core biopsy[25]. Local anaesthetic should be injected into the skin and deeply into the breast tissue around the target area. Local anaesthetic combined with adrenaline to promote vasoconstriction is recommended for infiltration of the breast tissue around the biopsy site. The vacuum itself also appears to assist haemostasis and should be used to aspirate any bleeding during the sampling procedure. Volumes of 10–15 ml of local anaesthetic can be safely used. Local anaesthetic without adrenaline may be preferred for the skin and in patients who have contraindications to the use of adrenaline. Longer-acting local anaesthetic may also be used around the biopsy site. However, there are no comparative studies to show that this more complicated local anaesthetic regimen provides any less patient morbidity than the use of a single local anaesthetic preparation.

As with all biopsy techniques, the patient

5

should be fully informed verbally and with written instructions about why the procedure is taking place, what it involves, what they will experience during the biopsy, how long it will take, what they will need to do afterwards and where they will receive the result. Because of the cutting action of the trocar anticoagulant, therapy is probably a relative contraindication to VAM compared to automated core biopsy[26].

In circumstances where it may be difficult at a later date to identify the site in the breast where the sample had been taken from, a marker should be placed in the biopsy cavity before the needle is removed. This can be a small metallic clip (e.g. Micromark™ clip) or gel pellets (e.g. Gel Mark™)[27]. The most common reason for marking the biopsy cavity is where it is likely that all the calcifications will have been removed during the biopsy procedure and subsequent localisation for surgery may be required. In these circumstances the gel pellets have the advantage of being easily visible with ultrasound, and localisation for surgery can be performed under ultrasound rather than X-ray guidance[28,29]. Displacement of calcifications at the time of biopsy has also been described and for this reason it may be wise to always place some kind of marker at the biopsy site where there is a high likelihood of subsequent surgical excision being required[30].

When the biopsy needle is removed from the breast, local compression should be applied continuously directly over the biopsy site as firmly as the patient can tolerate for 10–15 minutes. When there is no evidence of any bleeding, the skin entry site should be closed with an adhesive strip or skin adhesive; a skin suture is not required. After-care is the same as for automated core biopsy but it is advisable to also apply folded swabs directly over the biopsy site with a secure skin dressing held in place by a tight-fitting brassiere or wrap-around bandage. The patient should keep this on for 48 hours.

If a large amount of tissue has been removed, a wrap-around pressure bandage should be used. All dressings can be removed after 48 hours.

As with other biopsy procedures, patients are advised not to undertake any vigorous exercise; particularly using the arm on the side of the breast biopsied, for at least 24 hours. They should be given an instruction leaflet that explains the procedure that has been performed, what to do if bleeding occurs (apply manual pressure as applied at the time of the biopsy), advice on the use of analgesia, which is not normally required, and a contact telephone number for advice should problems arise.

Indications for VAM

Mammotomy, with its ability to sample larger volumes of breast tissue, has been shown to be more reliable in confirming that no frankly malignant change is present in association with conditions such as radial scar and ADH[18,31–33]. For the same reason re-biopsy rates are significantly less when VAM is used compared to conventional automated core biopsy[32,34]. However, despite the wider sampling achievable by mammotomy, until studies show that this technique is completely reliable in excluding associated malignancy, surgical excision is still recommended for definitive diagnosis in these circumstances[19,35–39].

The scar tissue around the surgical site in the conserved breast, particularly following radiotherapy, can be extremely hard and difficult to biopsy by conventional means when recurrence of malignancy is suspected. The mammotomy device with its motorised cutting trocar can be used successfully to obtain sufficient tissue to achieve a reliable diagnosis.

For malignant lesions, where ascertaining excision margins is fundamental to confirming adequate treatment, mammotomy must not be considered a therapeutic procedure[19,38]. Orientation of the piecemeal cores of tissue is difficult and it is impossible to ascertain with any degree of certainty whether adequate clearance of excision margins has been obtained. However, for some benign lesions, such as fibroadenoma, mammotomy can be used for therapeutic excision. Ultrasound guidance is ideal for this procedure, which is significantly more cost-effective and associated with less morbidity than surgical excision.

Indications for stereotactic VAM:

- very small cluster of microcalcifications that is likely to be difficult to sample with core biopsy
- cluster of calcifications at a site difficult to access with core biopsy
- conventional core biopsy failed to provide sufficient material for diagnosis
- indeterminate microcalcifications where it is likely that larger tissues volumes will be required for diagnosis.

VAM will understage disease less than half as often as will conventional core biopsy[12,14,16,40]. The difference is particularly marked in the understaging of ductal carcinoma in situ (DCIS). In a large review of core and VAM carried out by Reynolds, DCIS was found at surgery following a biopsy result. ADH was reported in 41% of core biopsies and only 15% of vacuum-assisted samples. Jackman and colleagues found that core biopsy underestimated the presence of invasive malignancy associated with DCIS in just over 20% of cases, while this was found in only 11% where VAM had been used for preoperative sampling[41]. A similar study reported by Rosenfield Darling found that VAM underestimated the presence of invasive disease in patients with DCIS in half the number compared to core biopsy (10% compared to 21%) and understaged DCIS in 19% compared to 40%[6,42,43].

VAM is ideal for sampling calcifications associated with papillary lesions as it allows for the whole lesion to be excised along with a rim of surrounding normal tissue[44,45]. Papillary lesions are often reported as indeterminate by pathologists and removal of the whole lesion and histological confirmation that the lesion is entirely benign can be achieved without the need for surgical biopsy.

Indications for ultrasound-guided Mammotome™ biopsy include the following:

- mammographically detected architectural distortion visible on ultrasound (differentiation of radial scar from malignant disease)
- focal and suspicious microcalcifications visible on ultrasound
- lesions too small for conventional core biopsy
- lesions too superficial or deep in the breast for conventional core biopsy
- previous failed conventional core biopsy
- further evaluation of core or fine-needle aspiration showing suspicious changes of uncertain malignant potential (e.g. ADH or lobular carcinoma in situ or radial scar)
- diagnosis of recurrent disease in patients treated by conservation surgery.
- abnormalities where wide sampling is considered important (e.g. mammographic asymmetric density with a non-specific ultrasound correlate)
- removal of benign lesions such as fibroadenoma as an alternative to surgery
- removal of axillary lymph nodes for diagnosis or as part of sentinel node biopsy.

The main advantages of VAM compared to automated core biopsy are that it requires only a single pass of the probe into the breast to obtain multiple cores of tissue, the cores are contiguous and circumferential and the tissue volume removed is considerably larger. VAM is also associated with significantly less morbidity than core biopsy – most women who have experienced both profess to prefer mammotomy. The main comparative disadvantages are its increased cost (at least 15 times more for consumables) and that it takes significantly longer to perform.

Ultrasound-guided mammotomy

The HH Mammotome device is light and easy to use (Fig. 5.2)[20,46,47]. An initial ultrasound scan is carried out to identify the best direction for access to the abnormality. Local anaesthetic is injected into the skin, the breast tissue down to the lesion and liberally inferior to and around the lesion itself. The local anaesthetic needle is used to identify the best direction and angle in which to insert the Mammotome™ probe. The probe is placed through a 2-mm skin incision under direct real-time ultrasound vision so that the biopsy notch lies immediately behind, and not through, the lesion. The relationship between the sampling notch and the lesion can easily be identified on the scan by manually moving the cutting trocar. Samples are obtained by incremental rotating of the probe through

various angles up to 90° on either side of the 12 o'clock horizontal position. The number of samples taken depends on the type and size of the abnormality. In a few cases there may be difficulty in advancing the probe to the required site through dense uncompressed breast tissue. In these circumstances, forming a track for the probe with the local anaesthetic injection is usually effective. Alternatively, a radiofrequency outer sheath can be placed for the mammotome probe to be passed through to the biopsy site. As the patient is lying supine, the procedure is well tolerated. Haematoma is kept to a minimum because the breast is not under compression and intermittent suction is applied through the probe at the biopsy site.

X-ray stereotactic-guided mammotomy

The techniques for prone table and upright VAM are very similar to those for conventional automated core biopsy[23,48]. Special attachments are needed for the probe guides and all manufacturers can provide these. The localisation software for the equipment must also be amended to allow for accurate place-

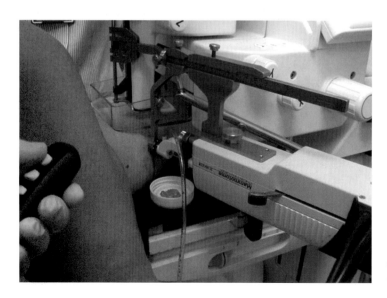

Fig. 5.6
The Mammotome ST™ in use with the GE Senovision™ system.

ment of the probe. The depth of passage is calculated as for core biopsy such that the centre of the sampling chamber corresponds to the point target selected on the stereoscopic images. VAM has been performed more widely on prone table devices but it is also easy to perform this technique on upright stereotactic devices using the Breast Care Ethicon Endosurgery Mammotome ST™ device. This has been designed for both prone and upright use (Figs 5.1 and 5.5). In the upright position, a lateral approach is preferred for most procedures as the probe is inserted in the long axis of the compressed breast (Figs 5.5 and 5.6). With this approach the compressed thickness of the breast is not a factor – with a vertical approach the compressed breast cannot be less than 30 mm or the sampling chamber will not be wholly within the breast and the vacuum will not function correctly. The lateral approach also allows for easier access to lesions lying superficially, close behind the nipple and close to the chest wall. These are all sites that can be difficult to target with core biopsy either with upright or prone biopsy tables[48].

Some concern has been expressed about possible long-term changes to the breast structure shown on mammography as a result of mammotomy but this has not been shown to be a particular problem[49]. Liberman et al. reported that immediate sequelae including air at the biopsy site and visible haematoma were common (72% and 60%, respectively) but that these changes resolve quickly leaving no long-term mammographic interpretation problems[50]. Similarly, Lamm and colleagues retrospectively reviewed 744 stereotactic core biopsies and found no abnormality at all in 96 of 225 vacuum-assisted mammotome procedures and only five mass lesions; in none of those with a residual abnormality did this cause any difficulty with mammographic interpretation[51]. Similarly, displacement of viable malignant cells by the vacuum-assisted technique is not

thought to be a significant problem[52,53].

Significant acute complications, mainly haematoma that requires intervention, are equally uncommon with VAM and core biopsy occurring in approximately 0.15% of cases[54]. Bruising following mammotomy is common for both procedures.

The contraindications to VAM are the same as those for conventional automated core biopsy.

Summary

VAM is a useful adjunct to core biopsy in the quest to achieve as high as possible non-operative diagnosis of breast calcifications. It is a flexible and accurate technique that can be used under both ultrasound and X-ray guidance. It provides the much larger tissue specimens needed by pathologists to make definitive diagnoses in borderline and other difficult cases and a method for the radiologist to obtain material from lesions that would otherwise be inaccessible to percutaneous biopsy. Despite the more accurate and reliable diagnoses achieved with VAM, the results should always be discussed in a multidisciplinary forum where the radiological and pathological concordance can be determined and the appropriate management discussed[37,55]. The main inhibition to the much wider use of VAM is the cost per case compared to conventional automated core biopsy[7].

References

1. Teh WL, Evans AJ, Wilson ARM. Definitive non-surgical breast diagnosis: the role of the radiologist. Clin Radiol 1998; 24: 11–9.
2. Parker SH, Burbank F, Jackman J et al. Percutaneous large-core breast biopsy: a multi-institutional study. Radiology 1994; 3: 359–63.
3. Vargas HI, Agbunag RV, Khaikhali I. State of the art of minimally invasive breast biopsy: principles and practice. Breast Cancer 2000; 7: 370–9.
4. Russin LD. New directions in breast biopsy: review

of current minimally invasive methods and presentation of a new coaxial technique. Semin Ultrasound CT MR 2000; 21: 395–403.

5. Parker SH, Burbank F. A practical approach to minimally invasive breast biopsy. Radiology 1996; 200: 11–20.

6. Darling ML, Smith DN, Lester SC et al. Atypical ductal hyperplasia and ductal carcinoma in situ as revealed by large-core needle breast biopsy: results of surgical excision. Am J Roentgenol 2000; 175: 1341–6.

7. Liberman L, Sama MP. Cost-effectiveness of stereotactic 11-gauge directional vacuum-assisted breast biopsy. Am J Roentgenol 2000; 175: 53–8.

8. Ferzli GS, Hurwitz JB, Puza T, Van Vorst-Bilotti S. Advanced breast biopsy instrumentation (ABBI): a critique. J Am Coll Surg 1997; 185: 145–51.

9. Ferzli GS, Hurwitz JB. Initial experience with breast biopsy utilizing the advanced breast biopsy instrumentation (ABBI). Surg Endosc 1997; 11: 393–7.

10. Heywang-Kobrunner SH, Schaumloffel U, Viehweg P, Hofer H, Buchmann J, Lampe D. Minimally invasive stereotaxic vacuum core breast biopsy. Eur Radiol 1998; 8: 377–85.

11. Liberman L, Dershaw DD, Rosen PP, Morris EA, Abramson AF, Borgen PI. Percutaneous removal of malignant mammographic lesions at stereotactic vacuum-assisted biopsy. Radiology 1998; 206: 711–15.

12. Burbank F. Stereotactic breast biopsy of atypical ductal hyperplasia and ductal carcinoma in situ lesions: improved accuracy with directional, vacuum-assisted biopsy. Radiology 1997; 202: 843–7.

13. Michell MJ, Andrews DA, Humphreys SEA. Results of 14-gauge biopsy of architectural distortion stellate lesions using a dedicated prone biopsy system. Breast 1996; 5: 442.

14. Jackman RJ, Nowels KW, Shepard MJ, Finkelstein SI, Marzoni F Jr. Stereotactic large-core needle biopsy of 450 non-palpable breast lesions with surgical correlation in lesions with cancer or atypical hyperplasia. Radiology 1994; 193: 91–5.

15. Liberman L, Cohen MA, Dershaw DD et al. Atypical ductal hyperplasia diagnosed at stereotaxic core biopsy of breast lesions: an indication for surgical biopsy. Am J Roentgenol 1995; 164: 1111–13.

16. Jackman RJ, Burbank F, Parker SH et al. Atypical ductal hyperplasia diagnosed at stereotactic breast biopsy: improved reliability with 14-guage, directional, vacuum-assisted biopsy. Radiology 1997; 204: 485–8.

17. Reynolds HE. Core biopsy of challenging benign breast conditions: a comprehensive literature review. Am J Roentgenol 2000; 174: 1245–50.

18. Brem RF, Schoonjans JM, Sanow L, Gatewood OM. Reliability of histologic diagnosis of breast cancer with stereotactic vacuum-assisted biopsy. Am Surg 2001; 67: 388–92.

19. Gajdos C, Levy M, Herman Z, Herman G, Bleiweiss IJ, Tartter PI. Complete removal of non-palpable breast malignancies with a stereotactic percutaneous vacuum-assisted biopsy instrument. J Am Coll Surg 1999; 189: 237–40.

20. Parker SH, Klaus AJ, McWey PJ et al. Sonographically guided directional vacuum-assisted breast biopsy using a handheld device. Am J Roentgenol 2001; 177: 405–8.

21. Parker SH, Dennis MA, Stavros AT, Johnson KK. A new breast biopsy technique. J Diagn Med Sonogr 1996; 12: 113–18.

22. Parker SH, Jobe WE, Dennis MA et al. US-guided automated large-core breast biopsy. Radiology 1997; 187: 507–11.

23. Parker SH, Klaus AJ. Performing a breast biopsy with a directional, vacuum-assisted biopsy instrument. Radiographics 1997; 17: 1233–52.

24. Brem RF, Schoonjans JM, Goodman SN, Nolten A, Askin FB, Gatewood OM. Non-palpable breast cancer: percutaneous diagnosis with 11-gauge and 8-gauge stereotactic vacuum-assisted biopsy devices. Radiology 2001; 219: 793–6.

25. Brem RF, Schoonjans JM. Local anesthesia in stereotactic, vacuum-assisted breast biopsy. Breast 2001; 7: 72–3.

26. Melotti MK, Berg WA. Core needle breast biopsy in patients undergoing anticoagulation therapy: preliminary results. Am J Roentgenol 2000; 174: 245–9.

27. Liberman L, Dershaw DD, Morris EA, Abramson AF, Thornton CM, Rosen PP. Clip placement after stereotactic vacuum-assisted breast biopsy. Radiology 1997; 205: 417–22.

28. Burbank F, Forcier N. Tissue marking clip for stereotactic breast biopsy: initial placement accuracy, long-term stability, and usefulness as a guide for wire localisation. Radiology 1997; 205: 407–15.

29. Parker SH, Kaske TI, Gerharter JE, Dennis MA, Chavez JL. Placement accuracy and ultrasonographic visualization of a new percutaneous breast biopsy marker. Radiology 2001; 221 (supplement): 431.

30. Lee SG, Piccoli CW, Hughes JS. Displacement of microcalcifications during stereotactic 11-gauge directional vacuum-assisted biopsy with marking clip placement: case report. Radiology 2001; 219: 495–7.

31. Philpotts LE, Shaheen NA, Carter D, Lange RC, Lee CH. Comparison of rebiopsy rates after stereotactic core needle biopsy of the breast with 11-gauge vacuum suction probe versus 14-gauge needle and automatic gun. Am J Roentgenol 1999; 172: 683–7.

32. Liberman L, Gougoutas CA, Zakowski MF et al.

5

Calcifications highly suggestive of malignancy: comparison of breast biopsy methods. Am J Roentgenol 2001; 177: 165–72.

33. Reynolds HE, Poon CM, Goulet RJ, Lazaridis CL. Biopsy of breast microcalcifications using an 11-gauge directional vacuum-assisted device. Am J Roentgenol 1998; 171: 611–13.

34. Liberman L, Smolkin JH, Dershaw DD, Morris EA, Abramson AF, Rosen PP. Calcification retrieval at stereotactic, 11-gauge, directional, vacuum-assisted breast biopsy. Radiology 1998; 208: 251–60.

35. Philpotts LE, Lee CH, Horvath LJ, Lange RC, Carter D, Tocino I. Underestimation of breast cancer with 11-gauge vacuum suction biopsy. Am J Roentgenol 2000; 175: 1047–50.

36. Cangiarella J, Gross J, Symmans WF et al. The incidence of positive margins with breast conserving therapy following mammotome biopsy for microcalcification. J Surg Oncol 2000; 74: 263–6.

37. Liberman L. Clinical management issues in percutaneous core breast biopsy. Radiol Clin North Am 2000; 38: 791–807.

38. Liberman L, Zakowski MF, Avery S et al. Complete percutaneous excision of infiltrating carcinoma at stereotactic breast biopsy: how can tumour size be assessed? Am J Roentgenol 1999; 173: 1315–22.

39. Won B, Reynolds HE, Lazaridis CL, P. JV. Stereotactic biopsy of ductal carcinoma in situ of the breast using an 11-gauge vacuum-assisted device: persistent underestimation of disease. Am J Roentgenol 1999; 173: 227–9.

40. Lee CH, Carter D, Philpotts LE et al. Ductal carcinoma in situ diagnosed with stereotactic core needle biopsy: can invasion be predicted? Radiology 2000; 217: 466–70.

41. Jackman RJ, Burbank F, Parker SH et al. Stereotactic breast biopsy of non-palpable lesions: determinants of ductal carcinoma in situ underestimation rates. Radiology 2001; 218: 497–502.

42. Burak WEJ, Owens KE, Tighe MB et al. Vacuum-assisted stereotactic breast biopsy: histologic underestimation of malignant lesions. Arch Surg 2000; 135: 700–3.

43. Brem R, Berndt V, Sanow L, Gatewood D. Atypical ductal hyperplasia: histological underestimation of carcinoma in tissue harvested from impalpable breast lesions using 11-guage stereotactically guided directional vacuum-assisted biopsy. Am J Roentgenol 1999; 172: 1405–7.

44. Guenin MA. Benign intraductal papilloma: diagnosis and removal at stereotactic vacuum-assisted directional biopsy guided by galactography. Radiology 2001; 218: 576–9.

45. Dennis MA, Parker S, Kaske TI, Stavros AT, Camp J. Incidental treatment of nipple discharge caused by benign intraductal papilloma through diagnostic mammotome biopsy. Am J Roentgenol 2000; 174: 1263–8.

46. Wilson ARM, Teh W. Mini symposium: imaging of the breast. Ultrasound of the breast. Imaging 1998; 9: 169–85.

47. Simon JR, Kalbhen CL, Cooper RA, Flisak ME. Accuracy and complication rates of US-guided vacuum-assisted core breast biopsy: initial results. Radiology 2000; 215: 694–7.

48. Nisbet AP, Borthwick-Clarke A, Scott N. 11-Gauge vacuum-assisted directional biopsy of breast calcifications, using upright stereotactic guidance. Eur J Radiol 2000; 36: 144–6.

49. Burbank F. Mammographic findings after 14-gauge automated needle and 14-gauge directional, vacuum-assisted stereotactic breast biopsies. Radiology 1997; 204: 153–6.

50. Liberman L, Hann LE, Dershaw DD, Morris EA, Abramson AF, Rosen PP. Mammographic findings after stereotactic 14-gauge vacuum biopsy. Radiology 1997; 203: 343–7.

51. Lamm RL, Jackman RJ. Mammographic abnormalities caused by percutaneous stereotactic biopsy of histologically benign lesions evident on follow-up mammograms. Am J Roentgenol 2000; 174: 753–6.

52. Diaz LK, Wiley EL, Venta LA. Are malignant cells displaced by large-gauge needle core biopsy of the breast? Am J Roentgenol 1999; 173: 1303–13.

53. Liberman L, Vuolo M, Dershaw DD et al. Epithelial displacement after stereotactic 11-gauge directional vacuum-assisted breast biopsy. Am J Roentgenol 1999; 172: 677–81.

54. Lai JT, Burrowes P, MacGregor JH. Vacuum-assisted large-core breast biopsy: complications and their incidence. Can Assoc Radiol J 2000; 51: 232–6.

55. Liberman L, Drotman M, Morris EA et al. Imaging–histologic discordance at percutaneous breast biopsy. Cancer 2000; 89: 2538–46.

5

A practical approach to the reporting of percutaneous sampling of breast calcifications

Sarah E. Pinder and Ian O. Ellis

Introduction

Non-operative diagnosis is essential in breast screening assessment to avoid surgical resection of tissue for diagnosis, particularly of benign lesions. In the UK, up to the mid 1990s, FNAC was the method of choice but the more recent introduction of automated core biopsy guns has led to the increasing use of tissue biopsy. The role of either technique for obtaining a non-operative diagnosis in malignancy is to provide a definitive diagnosis with subsequent rapid referral for treatment. Definitive non-operative diagnosis of benign conditions is also useful, leading to prompt reassurance and discharge with return to routine screening. It is well recognised that the greatest diagnostic accuracy in the non-operative diagnosis of breast disease is achieved using a "triple approach"[1,2]. This utilises the results of imaging and clinical examination with FNAC and/or core biopsy and, when all three modalities agree, reaches a very high level of diagnostic accuracy (>99%)[3]. Similar level of accuracy can be obtained when clinical examination is non-contributory for impalpable lesions[4]. In the UK National Health Service Breast Screening Programme (NHSBSP), audit has identified improved performance for needle core biopsy[5] and updated guidelines recommend core biopsy rather than FNAC as more appropriate for the assessment of calcific lesions[6]. As described in Chapter 4, the use of core biopsy sampling has especial benefits in the diagnosis of mammographic calcific lesions.

Core biopsy

Histological assessment of core biopsies cannot be performed reliably in isolation. The clinical and mammographic findings are vital for full evaluation, including the nature of the lesion and the site of sampling. If the core biopsy has been sampled from an area of calcification, multidisciplinary discussion and specimen X-ray are essential.

Calcification in core biopsy

After biopsies from mammographic microcalcifications have been X-rayed to determine whether calcium is present, they should be sent, ideally with a radiological comment regarding the presence or absence of representative microcalcification, to the histopathology laboratory along with the core sample. The specimen X-ray allows the pathologist to determine, not only the site of the calcification for which they are searching, but also the amount.

Examination of several levels (usually three) is performed initially, and if the calcification is not immediately apparent, further sections can be undertaken. It may be helpful for the cores in which the microcalcification is detected to be marked with a vital dye or sent to the laboratory in a separate specimen pot allowing "targeted" examination by deeper levels etc. should calcification not be detected in the initial series of sections. Thus comparison with the core biopsy X-ray allows the pathologist to concentrate on the particular core or portion of the sample that bears the calcification. On occasion, although calcification has been seen in the initial levels, it is clear from specimen X-ray that the amount is not representative of that present in the core and further levels may helpfully be examined.

Once the core biopsy has been X-rayed it should be placed immediately in fixative solution and sent promptly to the laboratory. Optimal fixation is paramount no matter what the nature of the lesion and ideally biopsies should be fixed for a minimum of 6 hours. After processing, routine haematoxylin and eosin (H&E)-stained sections are produced in the laboratory. Calcium takes different forms and has varying histological

6

appearances. For example, most calcifications have a haematoxyphilic nature and can be clearly seen with a deep purple colour on H&E sections. Calcium oxalate crystals, conversely, do not take up H&E stain and are often indistinct on routine sections but have a characteristic birefringence and rhomboidal structure when viewed with polarized light; further histochemical stains are therefore not in general required.

Diagnostic classification of core biopsies

Histological examination of core biopsy provides definitive diagnosis more often than FNAC[7] but it is important to recognise that it is not always possible to give an unequivocal diagnosis in all cases, although this is possible in the majority (> 90%). Most core biopsy samples can be classified as normal, benign or malignant but a small proportion of samples cannot. Some difficult cases may require further sectioning and, in problematic cases, histochemical and immunohistochemical studies may be helpful. Because of this and because of the requirements for fixation and processing, immediate reporting of core

biopsy is not possible, in contrast to FNAC where a result may be available rapidly and within less than 1 hour.

Core categories

B1 – normal

A core sample composed entirely of normal tissue is classified as B1, whether or not breast epithelial structures are present. Thus a sample of normal breast ducts and lobules or mature adipose tissue or stroma alone is categorised as B1. This may indicate that the lesion has not been sampled but this is not necessarily the case. Some benign lesions such as hamartomas and lipomas will provide normal histological features on core biopsy.

Normal breast cores may contain microcalcification, for example within stroma (Fig. 6.1) or in involutional lobules. It is essential that these cases be discussed in a multidisciplinary forum to confirm the appropriateness of the microcalcification in the histological specimen. Small foci of calcification within involuted lobules are common and may be too small to be visible mammographically although they are evident microscopically (Fig. 6.2).

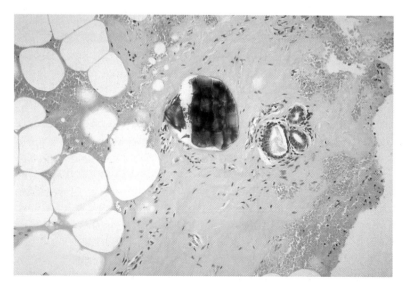

Fig. 6.1
Histological image showing calcification of normal breast stroma.

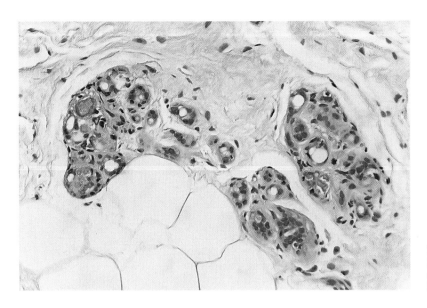

Fig. 6.2
Histological image showing calcification within atrophic lobules.

Microcalcification, either singly or in clusters less than 100 µm in diameter, is not visible radiologically[8]. A histological report that merely notes the presence of this calcification without additional comment on its nature, size and site is unhelpful, may be misleading and can lead to false reassurance and delay in diagnosis.

B2 – benign

A core biopsy sample is classified as B2 when it contains a specific benign abnormality. Thus a range of benign lesions including fibroadenomas, fibrocystic changes, sclerosing adenosis and duct ectasia may contain calcification and will fall within the B2 category for core biopsy. This also extends to include other non-parenchymal lesions such as abscesses and fat necrosis (Fig. 6.3).

Calcification which is deemed representative of the mammographic lesion radiologically and which can be confirmed to be in a specific benign lesion, such as a hyalinised fibroadenoma or fibroadenomatoid hyperplasia[9], can provide reassurance and the patient can be advised that surgical excision is not necessary unless they wish to have the lesion removed. A benign diagnosis from a calcific lesion in the absence of histological calcification, however, may not be considered sufficient and repeat sampling should be considered.

B3 – of uncertain malignant potential

This category is used for lesions which have benign histological features in the core biopsy sample, but the type of lesion identified is known in a proportion of cases to show heterogeneity with co-existing malignancy or to have an increased risk (albeit low) of associated malignancy. Thus included under the B3 category are atypical epithelial hyperplastic lesions where a uniform population of cells involves one duct space or only partially involves two or more duct spaces. These appearances raise the possibility of low grade DCIS but are insufficient in the tissue available to fulfil the diagnostic criteria (see also Chapter 2, Intraductal epithelial lesions)[10]. There is a range of degree, from those which are insufficient for a definite diagnosis of DCIS but highly suspicious, to those which only show minor degrees of atypia which requires further

6

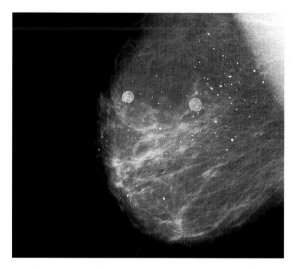

Fig. 6.3
A mammographic image following previous excision of a benign abnormality. Widespread punctate calcifications are demonstrated due to fat necrosis; in addition, calcified oil cysts are seen.

assessment. Appropriate categorisation into B3 or B4 is undertaken by the pathologist based on the degree of suspicion.

The definition of ADH relies on a combination of histological and morphological features and extent of disease and it is essentially an intraductal epithelial proliferation showing the features of low grade DCIS but in less than two duct spaces or less than 2 mm in diameter. For this reason, accurate diagnosis of ADH is not possible on core biopsy. Series of subsequent surgical diagnoses in cases described as ADH in non-operative core biopsy show that in over 50% the surgical excision biopsy has contained either in situ or invasive carcinoma[11]. This is not surprising as the limited tissue sampling that can be undertaken by core biopsy guns (often by stereotactic methods for foci of microcalcification) often provides insufficient material for definitive diagnosis of low grade DCIS. As described in Chapter 2, a greater number of cores particular bearing increased number of calcifications[12] or larger bore samples (such as the Mammotome™ device, see Chapter 5) may be helpful.

A proportion, usually of larger, radial scars/complex sclerosing lesions are now recognised to harbour forms of breast carcinoma often in the form of low grade DCIS or invasive tubular cancer. Papillomas, again usually the larger forms, can be heterogeneous and have focal areas of in situ carcinoma. In addition, categorical distinction between benign papillomas and papillary carcinomas in situ can be problematic in small tissue samples. Thus similar principles apply to lesions such as radial scars/complex sclerosing lesions and to papillomas (all of which may have associated microcalcification) sampled by core biopsy as apply to core biopsies bearing ADH. Unless the lesion has been very widely sampled by multiple core biopsies, or removed by mammotomy, current guidelines recommend classification of these lesions as B3.

A wide variety of rare lesions, which rarely contain calcification, such as phyllodes tumour and spindle cell proliferation, can present mammographically and a confident diagnosis cannot be achieved on routine core biopsy. In such circumstances we recommend that these are also classified as B3 and advise diagnostic surgical excision.

B4 – suspicious

Rarely, apparently neoplastic cells are contained within blood clot or adherent to the outer aspect of the sample and these are classified as B4 suspicious. Very small foci of invasive carcinoma, in which there is insufficient material to allow immunocytochemical studies, may also on occasions be assigned to this category.

A single complete duct space bearing an unequivocal high grade malignant epithelial proliferation is classified as B5 malignant and the features are those of high grade DCIS. Care is, however, taken if one or only part of a duct space is seen containing a highly atypical epithelial process (particularly if no necrosis is present); this may be regarded as suspicious rather than definitively malignant. Care is essential if the epithelial cells show apocrine features as this may represent an atypical apocrine proliferation but not apocrine DCIS.

Another lesion, which may be derived from mammographic calcification, and which must on occasion be classified as suspicious rather than malignant, is a non-high grade intraductal proliferation with a significant degree of atypia which could represent intermediate- or low grade DCIS. Particular care is taken when relatively few involved duct spaces are represented in the biopsy. If there is doubt in the mind of the pathologist, and the number of ducts provided is sparse, they should take a pragmatic approach and report an atypical intraductal proliferation, qualifying this according to the degree of suspicion. On the basis of extent or severity of atypia the core biopsy report is allocated to either the B3 or to B4 category. The management of cases classified as B3 or B4 will usually be either diagnostic excision biopsy of the area or repeat core or wider bore needle biopsy sampling to obtain definitive diagnosis. Multidisciplinary discussion is essential to ascertain what course of action is most appropriate for each individual case. In some cases it may be felt by the pathologist that the limited sampling available even with wide-bore needle sampling, may not provide sufficient material for reliable diagnosis and open biopsy may be more appropriate. The UK NHSBSP Non-Operative Guidelines note that definitive therapeutic surgery should not be undertaken as a result of a B3 or B4 core biopsy diagnosis[16].

B5 – malignant

The B5 category is used for cases of unequivocal malignancy on core biopsy. Further categorisation into in situ and invasive malignancy is undertaken whenever possible. One of the benefits of core biopsy is that it can allow distinction between in situ and invasive carcinoma, which is not possible on FNAC. Clearly, due to sampling error, presence of DCIS alone in the core does not exclude the presence of an invasive focus in the lesion, and in a proportion of cases sampled by standard methods, co-existing invasive carcinoma will be identified in the subsequent surgical excision specimen[13,14]. Conversely, invasive mammary carcinoma can be unequivocally identified in core biopsy with a positive predictive value of 98%[14].

The nuclear grade, architecture and the presence of necrosis of the DCIS can be indicated on the core biopsy report. The grade of DCIS on core biopsy correlates with subsequent grade of DCIS in the excision sample and also provides some limited assistance in the prediction of which cases may have a small associated invasive focus[13]. Many of these cores will derive from screen-detected microcalcifications and the presence of associated calcification should clearly be noted in the histological report. The site of the calcification should also be recorded, whilst in the majority microcalcification will be present

6

within the necrotic debris of the DCIS (Fig. 6.4); in some cases there may also be benign calcification in a co-existing benign process. The mammographic features can be reassessed in view of this data and the size of the malignant process re-evaluated.

FNAC

It is clear that FNAC is not the "gold standard" diagnostic technique; false positive cytology will occur. In particular it is important to note that certain lesions classified histologically as benign have malignant cytological features. These are generally borderline hyperplastic lesions, such as atypical hyperplasia. Histological diagnosis in these cases relies on cytomorphology but also extent and purity of the changes present and these are clearly not demonstrable in cytological preparations. Although ideally a definitive diagnosis of malignancy or benignity can be made on the majority of FNAC samples, the proportion where this is possible will increase with experience of both the pathologist and aspirator. If the sample is paucicellular or if the preparation is sub-optimal a clear distinction may not be possible.

Calcification in FNAC

FNAC from mammographically detected foci of calcification may be classified into any of the five diagnostic cytological categories recommended in the UK NHSBSP and it is of vital importance that the significance of each is understood in the multidisciplinary context. It is essential that the pathologist comments on the presence of calcification within the sample. If calcification is present, the radiologist and the multidisciplinary team can be more certain that the lesion has been sampled accurately and the likelihood of a false negative due to an aspiration miss is lower. It is important to note, however, that the presence of calcification in an FNAC from a calcific lesion does not discriminate between benign and malignant conditions and that the background cytological features are paramount.

FNAC categories

C1 – inadequate

The designation of an aspirate as "inadequate" is somewhat subjective. It is generally

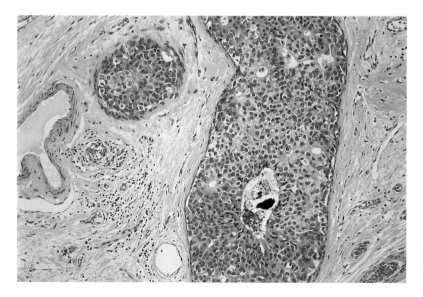

Fig. 6.4
Histological image showing a pleomorphic proliferation of intraductal epithelial cells with central necrosis and calcification. The appearances are of high grade DCIS.

based on the presence of sufficient numbers of epithelial cells to provide a sample adequate for confident assessment. There are a number of reasons for categorising a smear as inadequate: the preparation may be hypocellular, poorly spread or stained or obscured by blood. Conversely, aspirates from certain lesions, such as cysts, abscesses, fat necrosis and nipple discharge specimens may not contain epithelial cells but are not classified as inadequate. It is extremely unusual for a smear to contain microcalcification but insufficient epithelial cells for assessment and if this occurs, repeat sampling procedure should be performed, preferably core biopsy or diagnostic open biopsy.

C2 – benign

A benign sample with no evidence of significant atypia or malignancy is categorised as benign. The aspirate is usually poorly to moderately cellular and consists largely of regular epithelial cells. The background is usually composed of naked nuclei. A positive diagnosis of specific conditions, for example fibroadenoma, fat necrosis, granulomatous mastitis, breast abscess or lymph node, may be suggested if sufficient specific features are present to establish the diagnosis. The presence of microcalcification in a benign FNAC is supportive that the lesion has been sampled.

C3 – atypia probably benign

A C3 aspirate will have characteristics of a benign smear with, in addition, certain features not commonly seen in benign aspirates. These could be nuclear pleomorphism, some loss of cellular cohesiveness, nuclear or cytoplasmic changes or increased cellularity. In our unit the commonest benign lesion producing a C3 FNA is a fibroadenoma. Other low-grade and in situ carcinomas may also

give such a result[15]. Calcification may be seen in these lesions. The presence of calcification in a C3 smear provides neither reassurance nor should it produce unease; whatever the radiological suspicion, repeat sampling or diagnostic biopsy should be performed on a C3 result.

C4 – suspicious of malignancy

This category is used for aspirates where there are atypical features such that the pathologist is almost certain that they come from a malignant lesion. Confident diagnosis cannot be made because the specimen is scanty, poorly preserved or poorly prepared but has features of malignancy or it may show some malignant features without overt malignant cells present. Alternatively the sample may have an overall benign pattern but with occasional cells showing distinct malignant features. As with C3 results, the commonest malignant lesions in this category are low grade or special type lesions and also DCIS[15]. Similarly, the presence of calcification is non-contributory to subsequent management; further investigation is required. Definitive surgery should not be performed on the basis of a C4 result[16].

C5 – malignant

A malignant smear is usually cellular with cells showing discohesion, increase in cell size and pleomorphism and thus is interpreted as unequivocally malignant. It is well recognised that DCIS presenting as mammographically detected microcalcification is often high grade. FNAC of high grade DCIS, in general, if adequately sampled, bears large characteristically malignant cells along with necrosis; in this situation confident diagnosis can often be made. Low grade DCIS is more difficult to diagnose on FNAC and may be impossible to definitively diagnose; these cases will not infrequently be categorised as suspicious (C4) rather than malignant (C5) due to the paucicellular nature and the lack of large, overtly malignant cells. It should also be remembered that DCIS and invasive carcinoma cannot be distinguished by cytology alone.

The most common cause of false negative cytological diagnosis is an aspiration miss. There are, however, types of carcinoma which, by their nature, may produce a false negative diagnosis. The most common of these are tubular and lobular type carcinomas.

References

1. Ellis IO, Galea MH, Locker A et al. Early experience in breast cancer screening: emphasis on development of protocols for triple assessment. Breast 1993; 2: 148–53.
2. Lamb J, Anderson TJ, Dixon MJ, Levack P. Role of fine-needle aspiration cytology in breast cancer screening. J Clin Pathol 1987; 40: 705–9.
3. Zajdela A, Chossein NA, Pillerton JP. The value of aspiration cytology in the diagnosis of breast cancer. Cancer 1975; 35: 499–506.
4. Azavedo E, Svane G, Auer G. Stereotactic fine needle biopsy in 2594 mammographically detected non-palpable lesions. Lancet 1989; 1 1033–5.
5. Britton PD, McCann J. Needle biopsy in the NHS breast screening programme 1996/7: how much and how accurate? Breast 1999; 8: 5–11.
6. Wilson R, Asbury D, Cooke J, Michell M, Patnick J, editors. Clinical Guidelines for Breast Cancer Screening Assessment. Sheffield: NHS Cancer Screening Programmes 2001.
7. Britton PD. Fine needle aspiration or core biopsy. Breast 1999; 8: 1–4.
8. Dahlstrom JE, Sutton S, Jain S. Histologic–radiologic correlation of mammographically detected microcalcification in stereotactic core biopsies. Am J Surg Pathol 1998; 22: 256–9.
9. Kamal M, Evans AJ, Denley H, Pinder SE, Ellis IO. Fibroadenomatoid hyperplasia: a cause of suspicious microcalcification on mammographic screening. Am J Roentgenol 1998; 171: 1331–4.
10. Coordinating Group for Breast Screening Pathology. Pathology Reporting in Breast Cancer Screening, 2nd edn. NHS BSP Publications No 3, 1995.
11. Liberman L, Cohen MA, Dershaw DD et al. Atypical ductal hyperplasia diagnosed at stereotaxic core biopsy of breast lesions: an indication for surgical biopsy. Am J Roentgenol 1995; 164: 1111–13.
12. Bagnall MJC, Evans AJ, Wilson ARM, Burrell HC, Pinder SE, Ellis IO. When have mammographic calcifications been adequately sampled at needle core biopsy? Clin Radiol 2000; 55: 548–53.
13. Bagnall MJC, Evans AJ, Wilson ARM et al. Predicting invasion in mammographically-detected microcalcification. Clin Radiol 2001; 10; 828–832.
14. Liberman L, Dershaw DD, Rosen PP et al. Stereotaxic core biopsy of breast carcinoma: accuracy at predicting invasion. Radiology 1995; 194: 379–81.
15. Deb RA, Matthews P, Elston CW, Ellis IO, Pinder SE. An audit of "equivocal" (C3) and "suspicious"(C4) categories in fine-needle aspiration cytology of the breast. Cytopathology 2001; 12; 219–26.
16. Coordinating Group for Breast Screening Pathology. Guidelines for Non-operative Diagnostic Procedures and Reporting in Breast Cancer Screening. Sheffield: NHS Cancer Screening Programmes, 2001.

6

Chapter

7

A practical approach to the radiological diagnosis of breast calcification

Andy Evans and Robin Wilson

Recall

The most important decision regarding the diagnosis of calcifications is whether the features of the calcifications on the screening mammogram warrant recall. If calcifications are recalled to assessment it is unusual for the calcifications not to be correctly diagnosed as benign or malignant. Factors that should be taken into account when deciding whether to recall are their morphology, the distribution of the calcifications and the cluster shape. Other important factors include period change and whether similar calcifications are seen elsewhere in the same or opposite breast. Clinical history and physical findings are occasionally important.

Number

There is no magic number of calcific flecks above which clusters should be recalled and below which clusters should not be recalled. Three granular calcifications in a ductal distribution warrants recall, where four or five punctate calcifications in a round cluster with similar calcific flecks scattered elsewhere within the ipsilateral and contralateral breast probably do not warrant recall. It should always be remembered that the smaller the cluster, the less characteristic the morphology is for DCIS.

Morphology

Judgement as to whether a calcification cluster's morphology warrants recall should be based on the most suspicious of the morphological features present. The presence of punctate, rounded, oval calcifications within the cluster does not necessarily indicate benignity if there are other calcifications with more worrying morphological features, such as granular, elongated rod or branching calcifications. Rounded calcifications with central lucency are a reliable indicator of benignity. Variations in the size, shape and density of the calcifications increase the suspicion of malignancy although such features are found in many benign clusters. If elongated rod-shaped calcifications are present, the differential diagnosis lies between DCIS and duct ectasia. Caution should be adopted before diagnosing duct ectasia if the calcifications are unilateral and especially if the calcifications are not retro areolar. High-grade DCIS can give rise to quite coarse calcification, which appears very similar to duct ectasia.

Distribution

If a ductal distribution is present, unless there are categorical features of duct ectasia, the calcifications should be recalled as the only other common cause of a ductal distribution of calcifications is DCIS.

Cluster shape

Most clusters of benign calcifications are round or oval, whereas the vast majority of DCIS clusters have an irregular or V-shaped cluster shape. It is, however, not uncommon for DCIS when the cluster is small to have a round or oval cluster shape and this is particularly so in cases of low- or intermediate-grade DCIS. A multiple lobular distribution of calcifications normally indicates fibrocystic change but occasionally a multilobular distribution of calcifications can be found in intermediate- or low-grade DCIS.

Period change

Increase and decrease in the number of calcifications present over time is a common feature of both benign and malignant calcifications. New or increasing calcifications are often benign and just because calcifications are new does not automatically mean that recall is required. Calcifications that are totally unchanged over a 3-year period are very unlikely to represent DCIS and recall would only be warranted if they were of particularly suspicious morphology. It must also be appreciated, however, that decreasing calcifications do not necessarily imply that they are benign. We have had one case of Paget's disease of the nipple where obvious comedo calcification was present on the previous mammogram but which had totally disappeared by the time the patient presented with Paget's disease. A recent paper has also demonstrated that a third of cases where indeterminate calcification disappear are associated with the development of invasive carcinoma.

Is calcification elsewhere?

If a small cluster of calcification is found it is very important to critically review the whole of the affected and the opposite breast. If, on review, similar calcifications are seen elsewhere within the affected and in the opposite breast and these calcifications have a similar morphology, it is almost certain that this represents fibrocystic change and recall should only occur if the initial cluster identified has more worrying morphological features than the other calcifications demonstrated.

History

The threshold for recalling calcifications should be lower in patients whose clinical history or findings raise the possibility of DCIS. Low-risk calcifications in patients with single duct nipple discharge warrant further investigation.

Assessment of microcalcifications

Magnification views

High-quality magnification views should always be obtained in the CC and lateral planes. We routinely use a magnification factor of 1.5. The use of magnification factors higher than this can lead to blurring and can therefore degrade the quality of the image. One of the most important reasons for doing magnification views is to look for sedimentation to confirm the presence of fibrocystic change. The "tea cup" appearance should be visible on the lateral view and the calcifications should be more difficult to see and have an ill-defined rounded morphology on the craniocaudal view. In cases of fibrocystic change, magnification views will often identify smaller but similar calcifications elsewhere within the breast. Magnification views in cases of DCIS will often reveal smaller additional calcifications within the cluster when compared with the standard mammographic views. The magnification of views are also helpful for confirming the suspicious morphological features and a ductal distribution in such calcifications. In cases of malignant calcification, the magnification views should also be used to assess lesion size. Accurate assessment of lesion size is obviously important in counselling patients as to whether they are suitable for breast-conserving surgery or not.

Ultrasound

Ultrasound is often useful in the further assessment of cases of microcalcification. This is especially true in cases where there is a dense mammographic background pattern. In this situation there will often be a mammographically occult, but ultrasound-visible, mass. Often this mass is smaller than the calcification cluster and may indicate an invasive focus. Ultrasound-guided biopsy of invasive focus obviously benefits a patient as this will alert the surgeon to the need for an axillary staging procedure. Power Doppler examination of the area of microcalcification can sometimes show a focus of increased vascularity and this can also be helpful in guiding ultrasound-guided biopsy of an invasive focus. Ultrasound can also be helpful even in the absence of a mass as the calcifications can often be seen if high frequency 13 MHz probes are used[1]. In the absence of a mass, it is debatable whether ultrasound-guided core or stereotactic core biopsy should be performed. The results of ultrasound-guided core biopsy in the absence of a mammographic mass in this clinical setting tend to be slightly poorer than the results of stereotactic core if digital imaging is available.

Physical examination

Before image-guided biopsy is performed, it is important that the patient has a physical examination. A physical examination is helpful in identifying physical features associated with DCIS such as nipple discharge or Paget's disease. It is also important to know prior to biopsy whether the lesion is palpable and, if the lesion is shown to be malignant or suspicious on biopsy, one needs to know whether the lesion requires localisation or not. It is also helpful for the patient to meet the clinician who will give them the result of their biopsy prior to the receipt of the biopsy results.

Magnetic resonance imaging

Three studies of dynamic, contrast-enhanced MRI have shown that this imaging modality is both insensitive and non-specific in differentiating benign from malignant calcification clusters[2–4]. It is unclear whether DCIS assessment with MRI is superior to high-quality magnification views.

Scintimammography

Two studies have demonstrated that scintimammography in the clinical setting of mammographic microcalcification is relatively insensitive to in situ malignancy[4,5]. Its routine use in this clinical setting is therefore not advocated.

Biopsy – which technique?

The use of FNAC to biopsy mammographic microcalcification is not recommended as it is not possible to confirm representative sampling. The prefered choice of technique is whether to use core biopsy or a vacuum-assisted device. The main advantages of core biopsy are low cost and speed. The disadvantages are a lower calcification yield than mammotomy, difficulty in sampling calcifications behind the nipple and widespread diffuse clusters. Core biopsy is also more likely to understage DCIS and invasive cancer, yielding ADH results in cases of DCIS and DCIS results in cases that have an invasive focus. Repeat biopsies are more common following core than following mammotomy. The advantages of mammotomy are the increased calcification retrieval and less understaging of DCIS and invasive carcinoma[6]. The disadvantages of mammotomy are the cost of the disposables and lengthened procedure when compared with core biopsy. Core biopsy is, however, able to accurately diagnose a majority of calcification clusters and, for calcification clusters with 10 or more flecks in a tight cluster, the chances of diagnostic success are high. We would advocate the use of the mammotomy for small clusters, in cases of diffuse calcification and in calcification in the retro areola or inferior breast. Repeat biopsies should normally be performed by mammotomy. The major complications for mammotomy and core biopsy are identical at 0.1%.

7

Repeat biopsies

Repeat stereotactic biopsies are often helpful in patients with microcalcification[7]. If a benign result is obtained but no calcification is present on the specimen X-ray, a repeat biopsy is indicated. If a benign result is obtained and only one or two flecks of calcification were seen on specimen X-ray, a repeat biopsy is also likely to be required as false negative biopsies can occur in these circumstances[8]. A benign core biopsy and at least three flecks of calcification on the specimen X-ray indicate the patient can be discharged to routine follow-up unless the calcifications demonstrated are highly suspicious of malignancy, in which case a repeat percutaneous biopsy or surgical biopsy should be performed. In patients where the result of the needle biopsy is ADH, lobular carcinoma in situ or suspicious of DCIS, a repeat biopsy should normally be performed. Such decisions should be made at a multidisciplinary meeting where the pathologists and surgeon are present and this meeting should occur before the patient has been given the results of the biopsy. We rarely perform more than two percutaneous biopsies. If two biopsies are non-diagnostic, a surgical diagnostic biopsy should be performed. If a calcification cluster has been adequately sampled and a benign result obtained, there is no need for short-term follow-up. It is our experience that women placed on short-term follow-up have a higher incidence of anxiety and depression compared with women who are discharged back to routine follow-up.

References

1. Teh WL, Wilson ARM, Evans AJ, Burrell HC, Pinder SE, Ellis IO. Ultrasound guided core biopsy of suspicous mammographic calcifications using high frequency and power Doppler ultrasound. Clin Radiol 2000; 55: 390–4.
2. Westerhof JP, Fische U, Moritz JD, Oestmann JW. MR imaging of mammographically detected clustered microcalcifications: is there any value? Radiology 1998; 207: 675–81.
3. Gilles R, Meunier M, Lcuidarme O et al. Clustered breast microcalcifications: evaluation by dynamic contrast-enhanced subtraction MRI. J Comp Assist Tomogr 1996; 20: 9–14.
4. Tiling R, Khalkhali I, Sommer H et al. Limited value of scintimammography and contrast-enhanced MRI in the evaluation of microcalcification detected by mammography. Nucl Med Commun 1998; 19: 55–62.
5. Vanoli C, Anronaco R, Giovanella L, Ceriani L, Sessa F, Fugazzola C. ^{99m}Tc-MIBI characterization of breast microcalcifications. Correlations with scintigraphic and histopathologic findings. Radiol Med 1999; 98: 19–25.
6. Jackman RJ, Burbank F, Parker SH et al. Stereotactic breast biopsy of non-palpable lesions: determinants of DCIS underestimation rates. Radiology 2001; 218: 497–502.
7. Dershaw DD, Morris EA, Liberman L, Abramson AF. Non-diagnostic stereotaxic core breast biopsy: results of rebiopsy. Radiology 1996; 198: 323–5.
8. Bagnall MJC, Evans AJ, Wilson ARM, Burrell HC, Pinder SE, Ellis IO. When have mammographic calcifications been adequately sampled at needle core biopsy? Clin Radiol 2000; 55: 548–53.

7

Chapter

8

Localising breast calcification

H. Burrell

Introduction

The majority of cases of DCIS regarded as suitable for breast-conserving surgery are impalpable and therefore require image-guided localisation. Diagnostic surgical biopsy is also needed for mammographically indeterminate microcalcifications where image-guided biopsy has failed to make a definitive diagnosis. This includes cases where it has not been possible to obtain a representative sample of microcalcification at image-guided core biopsy or where the pathology of the tissue obtained is equivocal or suspicious for malignancy.

Some clusters of microcalcification may be superficially located within a small breast. In these cases it may be sufficient to place a marker on the skin directly over the lesion. This can be done by placing a piece of lead shot on the skin directly over the lesion and securing it in position with a piece of adhesive tape. Lateral and craniocaudal mammograms are then performed to check the position of the lead shot relative to the cluster of microcalcifications. If the position is satisfactory, the site of the lead shot on the skin is marked with an "X" using indelible marker pen. The majority of clusters of microcalcifications do not, however, lie superficially within the breast and it is therefore necessary to localise the cluster using a marker device placed under image guidance.

The most commonly used technique for image-guided localisation involves the insertion of a hookwire into the area requiring excision. Other techniques include radio-isotope localisation of clinically occult breast lesions; the use of carbon granules will also be discussed. The imaging modalities available to guide insertion of the marker device are either ultrasound or mammography, usually using stereotaxis

Hookwire localisation

The ideal localisation device should be acceptable to the patient, easy to place, be secure in position from the time of placement until the time of surgery and facilitate accurate surgical excision while allowing a good cosmetic result. A number of different hookwires have been manufactured for localising clinically occult breast lesions (Fig. 8.1). A wire is inserted into the breast inside an introducing needle following local anaesthetic infiltration of the skin. When the tip of the needle has been accurately placed within the lesion, the needle is withdrawn, leaving the tip of the wire in position and the excess wire protruding through the skin. The tip of the wire then provides a three-dimensionally stable guide for the surgeon. The disadvantage of a flexible wire is that the surgeon has to follow the wire from the skin down to the lesion and therefore the surgical approach to the lesion is governed by the direction of wire insertion. A flexible wire may also be inadvertently cut at the time of surgery[1,2]. A curved-end wire has the advantage that it can be pulled back into the introducing needle and repositioned within the breast if necessary and, if the localisation needle is left in situ, this acts as a palpable, anchored guide facilitating surgery[3,4]. The ability to straighten out the curve and pull the wire back into the needle does, however, weaken the stability of the wire[5]. Hookwires that protrude from the side of the needle provide a rigid guide which can be palpated by the surgeon and have greater anchoring strength than the flexible springhook wire and the curved-end wire[6–8]. The Reidy breast localisation needle is flexible and has an X-shaped tip, which is palpable and stable within the breast[9]. Once deployed within the breast, the Reidy wire cannot be repositioned and some pathologists have had problems with its

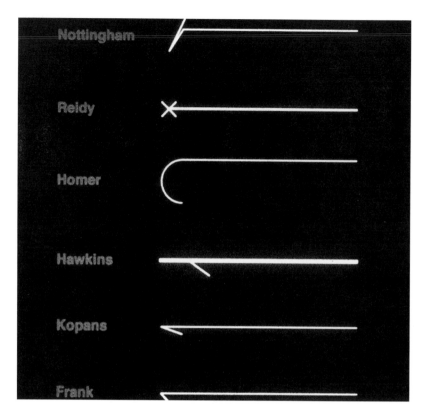

Fig. 8.1
Examples of various hookwires used to localise non-palpable breast lesions.

use as it can be difficult to remove from the surgical specimen without cutting into the tissue and interfering with specimen preparation[10]. The main disadvantage of leaving the introducing needle as well as the wire within the breast is the presence of the segment protruding through the skin. As this is not flexible, accidental trauma could result in tissue damage or displacement of the needle. This problem can be overcome by removing the localisation needle following insertion of the wire. At the time of surgery the surgeon can then place a blunt cannula over the wire until the tip of the cannula reaches the tip of the wire. The tip of the cannula is palpable and indicates the site of the lesion. The surgeon can then choose the optimal incision and route to the lesion allowing removal of the lesion with a good cosmetic result[10,11].

Ultrasound guidance

The proportion of clusters of microcalcification visible on high-frequency ultrasound varies from 52 to 93%[12–14]. This depends on a number of factors including the size of the cluster, depth of the cluster within the breast, presence of associated sonographic soft-tissue abnormalities and operator experience. For areas of microcalcification visible on high-frequency breast ultrasound, this is the method of choice for insertion of the marker wire. When using ultrasound, the technique is similar to that used for ultrasound-guided breast biopsy. The woman is in a supine oblique position with the ipsilateral arm elevated behind the head. The skin is infiltrated with local anaesthetic, and the introducing needle containing the wire is placed through the area of microcalcification using ultrasound guidance. The ideal position is for the wire to pass through the cluster with the tip lying just deep to it. The wire is inserted at an angle approximately 30° to the skin to avoid the potential complication of pneumothorax.

Stereotactic guidance

Whilst some have had success in recognising microcalcifications using very high-frequency probes (10–15 MHz[14]), many clusters are difficult to detect unless there is an associated soft-tissue abnormality. Localisation of microcalcification is therefore usually performed using stereotactic guidance. The direction of insertion of the localisation device depends on the location of the lesion within the breast and is chosen such that the wire traverses the minimum amount of breast tissue. When localising microcalcifications using stereotaxis, the accuracy of the procedure is dependent on choosing the same part of the cluster as the target on both stereotactic images. For lesions in the upper half of the breast, the wire should be inserted from above with the breast compressed in the craniocaudal position. For lesions in the lower outer quadrant, the wire is inserted from the lateral side, and for lesions in the lower inner quadrant, the wire is inserted from the medial side. The skin is infiltrated with local anaesthetic and the introducing needle containing the wire inserted through the cluster of microcalcifications. As with ultrasound localisation the ideal position is the wire traversing the microcalcifications with the tip of the wire immediately deep to the cluster. The potential difficulties of performing the procedure with upright stereotaxis such as patient movement and vasovagal attacks should be reduced by the use of digital technology as this significantly reduces the time taken to carry out the procedure.

Following both stereotactic and ultrasound localisation, the marker wire left protruding through the skin is covered in gauze and the gauze taped to the skin. The tip of the wire is fixed within the breast. The protruding wire is not taped to the skin in order that it is free to move in and out of the skin as the shape of the breast alters according to the woman's position. Cranio-caudal and lateral mammograms are then performed to check the position of the wire with respect to the lesion. The ideal position of the wire is such that it passes through the cluster of microcalcifications with the tip lying immediately deep to the lesion (Fig. 8.2). The position is adequate provided that the tip of the wire is within 10 mm of the lesion. Good communication between the radiologist and surgeon is vital. It is useful for the radiologist to provide a written description of the direction of insertion of the wire and its position in relation to the cluster of microcalcifications. The check mammograms demonstrating the wire position should be made available to the surgeon. If the tip of the wire is short of the lesion, the position is not adequate to guarantee successful surgical excision and the procedure will need to be repeated. Some of the hookwires such as the Nottingham wire can be removed by a firm tug. Others such as the Reidy wire cannot be removed except by surgical excision under anaesthesia and therefore, if the initial wire position is unsatisfactory, another wire should be inserted and the correct wire subsequently identified to the surgeon. The wire should remain stable within the breast, allowing surgery to be carried out later the same day.

Magnetic resonance imaging

Although there have been some reports stating that high-resolution magnetic resonance (MR) is able to visualise DCIS-induced microcalcification, most researchers cannot confirm this and MR has therefore no current role in the localisation of microcalcifications[15].

8

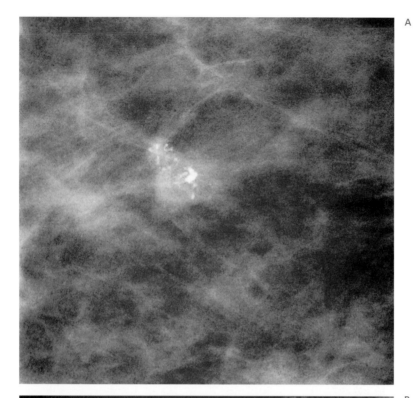

A

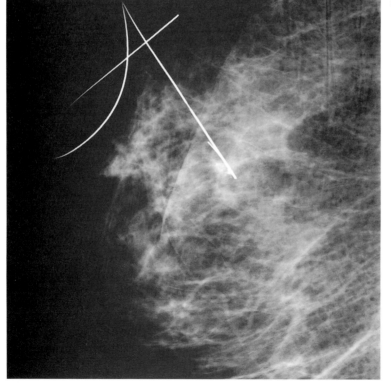

B

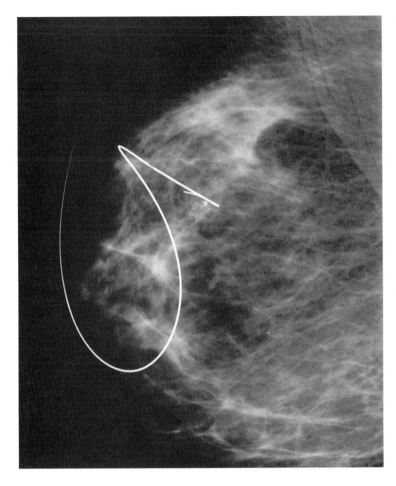

C

Fig. 8.2
(A) Magnification view of cluster of microcalcification. Stereotactic core biopsy demonstrated malignant calcification within an invasive carcinoma with mucinous features. (B) Lateral and (C) craniocaudal mammograms demonstrating the tip of the hookwire within the cluster of microcalcification.

Outcome and complications of hookwire localisation

The aim of the localisation procedure for non-palpable breast lesions is the removal of the suspicious lesion at the first surgical operation. The failure of excision rates published in the literature varies between 1.5% and 10%[10,16–21]. Some studies have shown that failure of localisation is more likely with microcalcifications than other mammographic lesions[22]. There are a number of possible reasons for failure to excise the mammographic lesion. These include the accuracy of the hookwire placement, experience and skill of the individual surgeon and migration of the wire within or out of the breast following placement and before surgery[22]. Migration of the wire is most likely to occur into the subcutaneous tissues with subsequent extrusion through the skin. Wires have, however, been reported to migrate some distance into the neck, axilla or even to the subcutaneous tissue of the buttock[23].

Other techniques

Use of dye and carbon

Preoperative marking of non-palpable breast lesions has been attempted using dyes such as methylene blue. Unfortunately the dye

8

119

tends to diffuse rapidly into the surrounding breast tissue and hence there is inaccuracy of marking even if the surgery is carried out within 4 hours of injection[24]. Carbon suspension as a marking medium was introduced in 1978 and has been widely used in some centres[25]. The non-palpable breast lesion is marked with a 4% aqueous suspension of carbon injected through a needle from the lesion out to the skin while the needle is being withdrawn. A black track of carbon particles is left within the breast and a tiny black point of carbon acts as a tattoo marking the site of injection in the skin. The carbon tract remains inert within the breast and the marking may therefore be performed days before surgery. At surgery, the surgeon dissects down the track to the lesion. Mullen et al. describe a 100% successful excision rate in

132 patients undergoing surgery following marking with carbon suspension[26]. In their series, the mammographic lesion underwent large-core needle biopsy using either a 14-gauge automated or 11-gauge vacuum-assisted device and, at the end of the biopsy procedure, the needle track was marked with carbon suspension injected through an 18-gauge needle. In the patients with a preoperative diagnosis of cancer there was no significant difference in the size of the surgical specimens with carbon marking compared with conventional hookwire localisation. No details were given regarding the adequacy of excision in these malignant cases. For the patients where localisation was performed for diagnostic purposes the mean size of the surgical specimen was 17 ml larger in the patients who had carbon marking

A

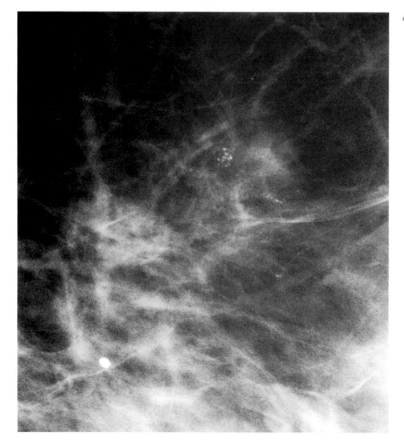

Fig. 8.3
(A) Magnification view of microcalcification due to intermediate grade ductal carcinoma in situ.

8

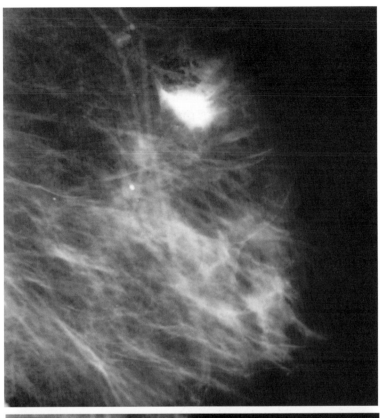

B

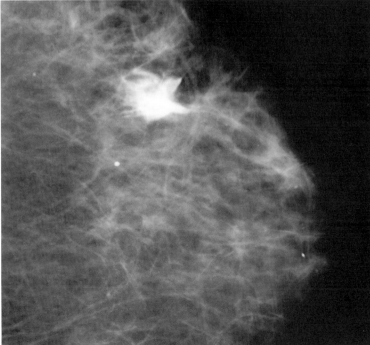

C

(B),(C) Lateral and craniocaudal mammograms following radiolabelled colloid localisation. The cluster of microcalcification is obscured by radio-opaque contrast medium indicating accurate localisation.

8

compared with hookwire localisation. The authors attributed this to the fact that the majority of these cases were performed during the learning curve phase early in the study. No difference was seen in the postsurgical cosmetic result. Carbon marking was well tolerated by the patients, did not create any mammographic abnormality and therefore did not interfere with subsequent mammographic follow-up. The main advantage of carbon marking is that it can be done at the time of the image-guided large-core biopsy and this avoids the need for a second procedure if the results of biopsy necessitate surgery. Needle seeding of cancer along the needle biopsy track has been described[27]. As the biopsy needle track is excised at the time of surgery following carbon marking, this is a potential advantage of this procedure compared with conventional hookwire localisation.

Radiolabelled colloid localisation

More recently, technetium-99m (^{99m}Tc)-labelled colloid albumin has been used for preoperative localisation of non-palpable breast lesions. Gennari et al. describe the technique in 647 patients[28]. In their series, 3.7 MBq (0.1 mCi) of ^{99m}Tc-labelled colloid particles of human serum albumin were injected into the non-palpable breast lesion using either stereotactic or ultrasound guidance. Frontal and lateral view planar scintigraphy images of the breast were obtained with a gamma camera immediately and 5 hours after administration of the ^{99m}Tc-labelled colloid particles. Superimposing these images on an appropriately enlarged mammogram checked the correct localisation of the tracer in the lesion. Surgical excision was carried out within 24 hours using a gamma-detecting probe to identify the area of maximum radioactivity corresponding to the site of the lesion. After excising the specimen, the probe was used to check for residual radioactivity at the excision site and if this was present the excision was enlarged. Subsequent radiography of the specimen verified the presence and centricity of the lesion in all but three patients (99.5%). In the remaining three patients, the lesion was successfully removed following a wider excision of tissue from around the 'hot spot' of radioactivity. The mean absorbed dose of radioactivity to the surgeons' hands from 100 such surgical procedures was estimated at 1% and 10% of the recommended annual dose limits for the general population and exposed workers, respectively. A comparison of radio-guided excision with wire localisation of occult breast lesions showed this new technique allowed a reduced excision volume with a better cosmetic result[29]. If a small volume (0.1–0.2 ml) of radio-opaque contrast medium is mixed with the radiolabelled colloid prior to injection, lateral and craniocaudal mammograms done immediately after the injection can be used to confirm accurate positioning of the radio-isotope in the mammographic lesion (Fig. 8.3). This obviates the need for scintigraphy[30].

Conclusion

In conclusion, microcalcifications can be successfully localised using a variety of techniques. The most commonly used method involves image-guided insertion of a hookwire. The use of carbon marking at the time of large-core needle biopsy avoids the need for a second procedure if surgery is required. An alternative technique using an injection of radiolabelled colloid has been shown to be as accurate and this may be more widely adopted in the future.

References

1. Hall FM, Frank HA. Preoperative localisation of non-palpable breast lesions. Am J Roentgenol 1979; 132: 101–5.

2. Kopans DB, DeLuca S. A modified needle-hookwire technique to simplify preoperative localization of occult breast lesions. Radiology 1980; 134: 781.

3. Homer MJ. Non-palpable breast lesion localization using a curved-end retractable wire. Radiology 1985; 157: 259–60.

4. Homer MJ. Localization of non-palpable breast lesions with the curved-end, retractable wire: leaving the needle in vivo. Am J Roentgenol 1988; 151: 919–20.

5. Kopans DB, Swann CA. Preoperative imaging-guided needle placement and localization of clinically occult breast lesions. Am J Roentgenol 1989; 152: 1–9.

6. Urratia EJ, Hawkins MC, Steinbach BG et al. Retractable-barb needle for breast lesion localization: use in 60 cases. Radiology 1988; 169: 845–7.

7. Walker TM, Ross HB. Localization of impalpable breast lesions using the Hawkins needle. Br J Radiol 1992; 65: 929–31.

8. Czarnecki DJ, Berridge DL, Splittgerber GF, Goell WS. Comparison of the anchoring strengths of the Kopans and Hawkins II needle-hookwire systems. Radiology 1992; 183: 573–4.

9. Chaudary MA, Reidy JF, Chaudhuri P, Millis RR, Hayward JL, Fentiman IS. Localisation of impalpable breast lesions: a new device. Br J Surg 1990; 77: 1191–2.

10. Burrell HC, Murphy CA, Wilson ARM et al. Wire localization biopsies of non-palpable breast lesions: the use of the Nottingham localization device. Breast 1997; 6: 79–83.

11. Kopans DB, Meyer JE. Versatile spring hookwire breast lesion localiser. Am J Roentgenol 1982; 138: 586–7.

12. Cilotti A, Bagnolesi P, Moretti M et al. Comparison of the diagnostic performance of high-frequency ultrasound as a first- or second-line diagnostic tool in non-palpable lesions of the breast. Eur Radiol 1997; 7: 1240–4.

13. Cleverley JR, Jackson AR, Bateman AC. Preoperative localisation of breast microcalcification using high-frequency ultrasound. Clin Radiol 1997; 52: 924–6.

14. Teh WL, Wilson ARM, Evans AJ, Burrell H, Pinder S, Ellis IO. Ultrasound-guided core biopsy of suspicious mammographic calcifications using high frequency and power Doppler ultrasound. Clin Radiol 2000; 55: 390–4.

15. Kuhl CK. MRI of breast tumors. Eur Radiol 2000; 10: 46–58.

16. Homer MJ. Localization of non-palpable breast lesions: technical aspects and analysis of 80 cases. Am J Roentgenol 1983; 140: 807–11.

17. Homer MJ, Pile-Spellmann ER. Needle localization of occult breast lesions with a curved-end retractable wire: technique and pitfalls. Radiology 1986; 161: 547–8.

18. Bigelow R, Smith R, Goodman PA, Wilson GS. Needle localization of non-palpable breast masses. Arch Surg 1985; 120: 565–9.

19. Gisvold JJ, Martin JK. Prebiopsy localization of nonpalpable breast lesions. Am J Roentgenol 1984; 143: 477–81.

20. Hall FM, Storella JM, Silverstone DZ, Wyshak G. Non-palpable breast lesions: recommendations for biopsy based on suspicion of carcinoma at mammography. Radiology 1988; 167: 353–8.

21. Tresadern JC, Ashbury D, Hartley G, Sellwood RA, Borg-Grech A, Watson RJ. Fine-wire localization and biopsy of non-palpable breast lesions. Br J Surg 1990; 77: 320–2.

22. Jackman RJ, Marzoni FA. Needle-localized breast biopsy: why do we fail? Radiology 1997; 204: 677–84.

23. Owen AWMC, Nanda Kumar E. Migration of localising wires used in guided biopsy of the breast. Clin Radiol 1991; 43: 251.

24. Svane G. A stereotaxic technique for preoperative marking of non-palpable breast lesions. Acta Radiol 1983; 24: 145–51.

25. Svane G. Stereotaxic needle biopsy of non-palpable breast lesions. A clinic–radiologic follow-up. Acta Radiol 1983; 24: 385–90.

26. Mullen DJ, Eisen RN, Newman RD, Perrone PM, Wilsey JC. The use of carbon marking after stereotactic large-core-needle breast biopsy. Radiology 2001; 218: 255–60.

27. Harter LP, Curtis JS, Ponto G et al. Malignant seeding of the needle tract during stereotaxic core needle breast biopsy. Radiology 1992; 185: 713–14.

28. Gennari RG, Galimberti V, De Cicco C et al. Use of technetium-99m-labeled colloid albumin for preoperative and intraoperative localization of non-palpable breast lesions. J Am Coll Surg 2000; 190: 692–9.

29. Luini A, Zurrida S, Paganelli G et al. Comparison of radioguided excision with wire localization of occult breast lesions. Br J Surg 1999; 86: 522–5.

30. Bagnall MJC, Rampaul R, Evans AJ, Wilson ARM, Burrell HC, Geraghty JG. Radio-guided occult lesion localization (ROLL) – a new method for locating impalpable breast lesions at surgery. Radiology 2000; 3 (IOS Supplement): 49.

8

Chapter

9

Clinical aspects of diagnosing microcalcification

R. D. Macmillan

Introduction

The large majority of breast lesions present-ing as microcalcification are impalpable. Their clinical management depends on his-tology and extent and is greatly facilitated, and possibly more effective, if a preoperative diagnosis can be made. Extensive areas of microcalcification rarely present a problem in this regard and, as almost all of those that are clinically significant will be extensive DCIS, management decisions are not difficult. Small, localised clusters of microcalcification may be less amenable to radiological biopsy and an open diagnostic biopsy may be required. When a preoperative diagnosis of malignancy has been made, therapeutic wide local excision may be appropriate. Excision of non-palpable lesions is now a relatively routine procedure for breast surgeons. The extent of surgery may be influenced by mam-mographic findings both for calcification associated with pure DCIS and also for microcalcification present within and around invasive lesions. Microcalcification may also be the presenting feature of non-malignant lesions that predict increased breast cancer risk. This chapter will discuss the clinical aspects of these issues.

Calcification and DCIS

The incidence of DCIS has increased sixfold over the past 15 years. The mode of presenta-tion has also changed from a palpable mass, nipple discharge or Paget's disease to the current situation in which approximately 90% of all DCIS cases present as clini-cally occult lesions on mammography. Approximately 80% of these are present as microcalcification. This is of course due to mammographic screening in which, for women aged 50–65, 20% of all cancers detected are DCIS. If younger women are screened, this percentage is reportedly as high as 40%.

The optimum management of DCIS is still debated. Uncertainty remains about which women should be treated by mastectomy and which by wide local excision. No ran-domised trial has ever compared wide local excision to mastectomy for the treatment of DCIS and, whilst mastectomy is virtually curative, a small but significant risk of local recurrence is reported by all series of wide local excision. Factors used to predict this risk include close pathological margin status, high-grade and comedo histological subtype. Scoring systems have been developed which weight these factors to predict risk of recur-rence and that proposed by the Van Nuys Group is perhaps the most widely used[1]. There is general agreement that margin status is of paramount importance. This is, of course, not available until an attempt at ther-apeutic surgery has been performed. In three randomised trials in which wide local exci-sion alone has been compared with adjuvant radiotherapy, local recurrence rates are significantly reduced by radiotherapy. However, it is clear that not all women require radiotherapy (indeed the large majority do not) and a few women will get local recurrence even after receiving it.

Several reports have assessed mammo-graphic appearances for predicting the likely success of breast-conserving surgery for DCIS. Only one study has used actual local recurrence rate as its primary outcome measure. This reported that proximity of microcalcifications to within 40 mm of the nipple was associated with increased risk of local recurrence[2]. The local recurrence rate at 5 years was 36.6% (11 of 46) in the close group compared to 12.8% (four of 83) in the distant group. In another study of 37 cases, risk of local recurrence (as predicted by the Van Nuys prognostic index) was lowest with fine granular microcalcifications, moderate with coarse granular microcalcifications and highest with linear branching microcalcifica-tions[3]. This was principally due to the

9

association between linear branching micro-calcifications, and to a lesser extent coarse granular calcification, with high nuclear grade. Linear pattern calcification, particularly if branching, is strongly associated with both nuclear grade and presence of comedo necrosis[4-8]. Of 198 cases of DCIS diagnosed in Kopparberg County, Sweden between 1977 and 1994, 151 (76%) presented as microcalcification[8]. The distribution of grade according to type of calcification is shown in Table 9.1.

What is the clinical relevance of being able to predict grade of DCIS by mammography? In both the NSABP and EORTC randomised trials of wide local excision for DCIS in which women were randomised to adjuvant radiotherapy or not, high-grade/comedo necrosis was a significant independent predictor of local recurrence risk[9,10]. In addition, invasive local recurrences in women with high-grade DCIS tend to be grade 3 cancers[11]. Hence mortality from invasive recurrences of DCIS, although small, is greatest in those who had high-grade DCIS. In the EORTC trial, 11 of the 14 women (79%) who developed metastases following an invasive local recurrence had originally been treated for high-grade DCIS[10]. Thus, if women with high-grade DCIS are to be treated by breast-conserving surgery, it is important that local treatment is adequate. Young women are more likely to have high-grade DCIS and it is this group who are perhaps most likely to chose breast-conserving surgery. Knowing preoperatively that a woman is likely to have high-grade

DCIS may influence the extent of surgical excision.

However, the DCIS collaborative group sounded a cautionary note regarding the significance of grade[12]. Although it significantly correlated with local recurrence at 5 years (12% versus 3%), at 10 years this correlation was all but lost (18% versus 15%). This would suggest that grade of DCIS might be a predictor of time to local recurrence as well as grade of invasive local recurrence.

Currently, mammographic extent of microcalcification rather than type of calcification is the main preoperative determinant of suitability for breast-conserving surgery. Discrepancy between this and pathological extent measured at microscopy is obviously of relevance. This was assessed by Holland et al.[13]; in a series of 82 mastectomy specimens, 47% of the micropapillary/cribriform DCIS type showed a discrepancy of greater than 20 mm between radiological and pathological extent compared to only 16% of comedo-type DCIS. However, in a later publication analysing a series of 35 cases, the relationship between discrepancy in size and type of DCIS was lost if magnification views of the calcification were performed[4]. This is now standard practice. However, despite magnification the pathological extent of 17% of all cases in this series was still underestimated by more that 2 cm.

Margin analysis of wide local excision specimens for DCIS is not, unfortunately, an exact science. Hence despite a widely held

Table 9.1 Distribution of grade according to type of calcification

	Linear	Coarse granular	Fine granular
No. of cases (%)	46 (30.5%)	78 (51.7%)	27 (17.9%)
High grade	37 (80.4%)	35 (44%)	3 (11.1%)
Low/Intermediate grade	9 (19.6%)	43 (55.1%)	24 (88.9%)

From Tabar et al.[8]

9

belief that DCIS is a contiguous disease process, all series of breast-conserving surgery report a rate of local recurrence despite apparently clear margins. This rate is higher if radiotherapy is omitted and affects the site of previous excision in approximately 80% of cases. The chance of achieving clear surgical margins is greatest at initial surgery, hence the importance of preoperative diagnosis. It can be difficult at re-operation to identify the original site of the lesion and histological interpretation of scarred and diathermised tissue can be problematic. In a recent analysis of the Nottingham DCIS series, 24/28 local recurrences (86%) occurred in women who had undergone re-excision to (apparently) clear margins after either diagnostic or initial therapeutic surgery[14]. The chance of clear margins is also greater, unsurprisingly, with increasing width of excision[15]. There is an argument perhaps for recommending a wider (2–3 cm) margin for high-grade DCIS (linear calcification) than for low-grade DCIS (fine granular calcification) and it may be that fewer cases of high-grade DCIS are suitable for breast-conserving surgery on the basis of this criteria alone.

Calcification and invasive cancer

Associated microcalcification also has significance for invasive lesions. It correlates with tumour grade, one study showing that it occurred with 31% of high-grade cancers compared to only 6% of low-grade cancers[16]. Six studies have shown that it correlates with an increased risk of involved surgical excision margins after wide local excision[17-22]. Two studies have reported that two-thirds of women who have cancers with associated calcifications have involved cavity wall shavings following wide local excision[17,18]. This is particularly likely with linear calcifications[17].

Beron et al. showed in a series of 190 patients that mammographic calcification of any sort was associated with an increased chance of finding residual disease at re-excision (35% versus 11% with no calcifications)[22]. In a study of 381 women, a stellate lesion with associated microcalcification was associated with a 3.8-fold (95% CI 1.1–13.0) increase in local recurrence[21].

Extensive in situ disease surrounding an invasive cancer is also recognised as a risk factor for local recurrence after wide local excision. Five-year local recurrence rates have been reported to be 3.5-fold higher in those with an EIC[23]. In 105 cases, Healey et al. showed that cancers with EIC were more likely to be associated with mammographic calcification than those without EIC (83% versus 27%)[24].

Absence of mammographic calcification surrounding an invasive ductal carcinoma may be the best predictor of unifocality[21]. Of 135 mastectomy specimens containing tumours < 4 cm (44% less than 2 cm), 90 had no associated calcification. Of these, 39% had multifocal disease beyond 1 cm from the dominant mass histologically compared to 62% in those with associated calcification. Surgeons should certainly take note of the presence and type of calcification within and around invasive cancers. Patients with microcalcifications may be selected for wider excision or in some cases may be deemed unsuitable for breast-conserving surgery and prospective studies assessing this, perhaps assessing the significance of different patterns of microcalcification, are required.

Certain types of microcalcification have even been proposed as having independently significant prognostic value[25]. In a retrospective study of 343 patients with breast cancers <15 mm, casting-type calcifications appeared to select a group of women with a poor prognosis. In view of the association between this feature and tumour grade, this is almost certainly a secondary prognostic variable and it is difficult to envisage its clinical utility.

Calcification and atypical hyperplasias

A relatively common reason for a diagnostic excision of microcalcification is ADH. Of all diagnostic excisions performed for a pre-operative diagnosis of ADH, 25–47% will be DCIS or invasive cancer[26–29]. One study suggested that mild ADH found on mammotome biopsy may not need surgical excision if all calcification was excised[30]. However, the main clinical difficulty encountered with ADH is the variability in pathological interpretation of this lesion between different pathologists. Nevertheless, surgical biopsy is necessary and, as ADH is commonly associated with malignant lesions, it may be appropriate to discuss therapeutic excision of the lesion as the first operative procedure (see below).

Wire-guided biopsy

For impalpable lesions the most common method of performing either diagnostic or therapeutic surgery is wire-guided biopsy. Other approaches are under investigation.

The surgical technique for both diagnostic and therapeutic wire-guided biopsy is similar, with the exception that a diagnostic operation is often *incisional*, the priority being to remove the minimal amount of tissue sufficient for diagnosis with maximal consideration for cosmesis. Accepting this principle it is still sometimes prudent to consent the patient for and intentionally perform a therapeutic excision for small lesions where the degree of radiological suspicion is high and the resultant additional effect on cosmesis is negligible.

In performing wire-guided surgery, the initial step is to make a spatial appraisal of the lesion from the mammograms in relation to its position within the breast, relationship to the nipple, skin and chest wall. The next step is to ascertain the full extent of the lesion, and inking of its perimeter on the mammograms by the radiologist may aid this. To this end, a magnification view of the microcalcification is essential. The final preoperative step is to determine the position of the lesion in relation to the tip of the wire. Ideally the wire tip should be within the lesion or just beyond it (Figs 9.1 and 9.2). Two-view mammography is required for this process and craniocaudal and true lateral films may be the ideal combination. Attention is then turned to the breast and placement of the surgical scar. This should be directly over the lesion. Minor adjustments to enhance cosmesis are acceptable but re-excision rates are high after both diagnostic and therapeutic procedures for microcalcification and second excisions are easier when the wound lies directly over the cavity. Most wire-guided localisation systems involve a rigid cannula being fed over a flexible guide wire. This should be performed with the wire straight. It thus needs to be held under slight tension and an assistant should manipulate the breast to approximate the position in which the wire was inserted (recorded by the radiologist), so straightening it. Once the rigid cannula is advanced to the tip of the wire, the site of the lesion is often easily palpable by balloting the tissue between the tip of the cannula and the overlying skin. This in turn is made easier if there is a relatively short length of cannula within the breast. At operation the position of the wire tip is repeatedly checked by balloting the cannula. When surgery is for an invasive cancer or when there is a mass lesion on mammography, there is often a palpable nodule intraoperatively, which can guide excision. This is not the case for DCIS presenting as microcalcification only, for which there is usually no palpable abnormality even intraoperatively.

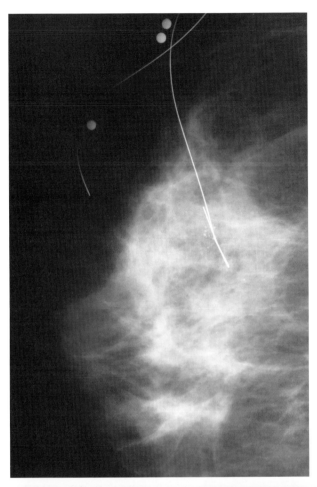

Fig. 9.1
Mammography following stereotactic localising wire insertion. This check image shows the tip of the wire just through the cluster of microcalcifications. This is the ideal wire position.

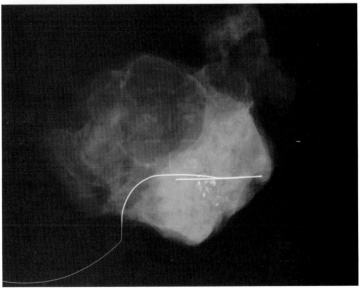

Fig. 9.2
Specimen X-ray on a diagnostic wire localisation showing adequate sampling of the calcification cluster.

The superficial plane of dissection over the lesion is initially dissected. In fatty breasts, which can "crumble" easily during surgery, great care needs to be taken to avoid displacement of the guide wire. For a therapeutic procedure, I then normally develop the planes of dissection parallel to the tip of the cannula, then dissect the margins distal and deep to the cannula tip before completing the excision by removing the cannula and dividing the wire at the desired margin of excision. The specimen is marked, X-rayed and margins of excision assessed (Fig. 9.3). Two-dimensional X-ray is appropriate if excision margins have not been taken to skin superficially and pectoral fascia deeply. Surgical clips left in the cavity may help to identify the site of the lesion if a re-excision is required.

With relatively large areas of microcalcification, or where it forms a more linear distribution, bracketing by two wires may be helpful. This can allow large lesions to be widely excised with cosmetic reshaping, reduction or volume replacement procedures.

Radio-guided biopsy

An alternative technique to wire-guided surgery is radio-occult lesion localisation (ROLL). This utilises ^{99m}Tc-labelled macromolecules to localise the lesion, which can then be detected using a gamma probe. The macromolecules do not migrate within the breast and are excised as part of the excision specimen. A check film is required to confirm correct placement of the marker. This can be achieved either by a scintigram or by injecting a small amount of radio-opaque dye with the macromolecules and confirming correct placement with a mammogram (Fig. 9.4). This technique has potential advantages over wire-guided biopsy. One advantage for surgeons is that the site of the lesion is readily identified throughout the operation and absence of radioactivity within the cavity confirms that the lesion lies within the specimen. It can be performed on the day or even the day before surgery and it is also not subject to displacement, unlike guide wires. One disadvantage encountered in the Nottingham series was that, for two patients,

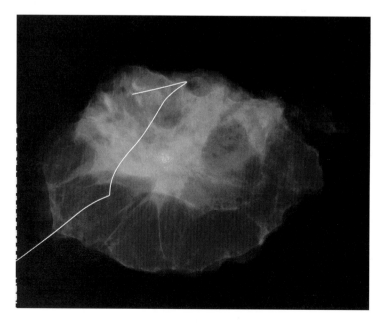

Fig. 9.3
Therapeutic wide local excision specimen X-ray showing the small cluster of microcalcifications representing DCIS centrally within the excision. Approximately 1–2 cm excision margin is seen radiologically.

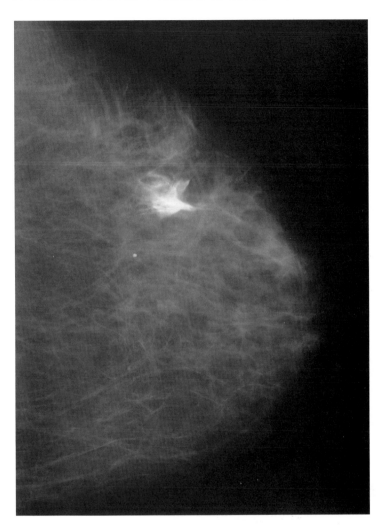

Fig. 9.4
Mammographic check film of ROLL. It can be seen that the injection of water-soluble ionic contrast media overlies a small cluster of microcalcifications.

the radio-opaque dye was inadvertently injected into a duct and the check mammogram revealed a galactogram appearance with diffuse radioactive uptake. Wire-guided biopsy was possible after allowing approximately an hour for the dye to clear (Fig. 9.5). In a comparison with wire-localisation, one study found that ROLL excision specimens were smaller and the lesion was better centred[31]. In a randomised trial comparing these procedures, ROLL was quicker and easier to perform. Accuracy of the two techniques was similar but patient satisfaction was higher with ROLL[32].

Conclusions

Clinically significant breast microcalcification has several implications for the management of premalignant and invasive breast lesions. It can give important clues as to the biology of the disease process and this information may currently be under-utilised in the preoperative decision-making process. For both DCIS and invasive breast cancer, associated microcalcification can indicate the need for wider excision and is strongly associated with grade. It should therefore be a consideration in the decision to recommend

9

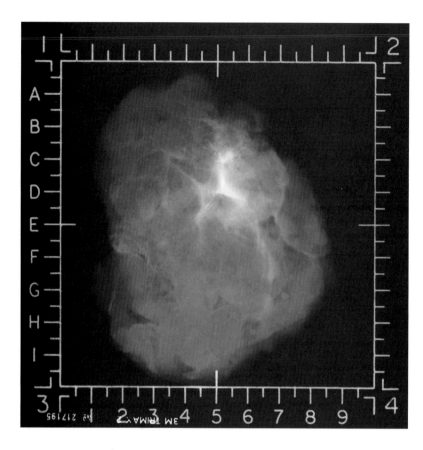

Fig. 9.5
Specimen X-ray following a ROLL therapeutic excision. Microcalcifications can be seen adjacent to residual ionic contrast.

breast-conserving surgery. Such surgery requires careful appreciation of the mammographic findings and ROLL may be a useful new technique to facilitate it.

References

1. Silverstein MJ, Lagios MD, Craig PH, Waisman JR, Lewinsky BS, Colburn WJ, Poller DN. A prognostic index for ductal carcinoma in situ of the breast. Cancer 1996; 77: 2267–74.
2. Stallard S, Hole DA, Purushotham AD et al. Ductal carcinoma in situ of the breast – among factors predicting for recurrence, distance from the nipple is important. Eur J Surg Oncol 2001; 27: 373–7.
3. Lee KS, Han BH, Chun YK, Kim HS, Kim EE. Correlation between mammographic manifestations and averaged histopathologic nuclear grade using prognosis–predict scoring system for the prognosis of ductal carcinoma in situ. Clin Imaging 1999; 23: 339–46.
4. Holland R, Hendriks JH. Microcalcifications associated with ductal carcinoma in situ: mammographic–pathologic correlation. Semin Diagn Pathol 1994; 11: 181–92.
5. Dinkel HP, Gassel AM, Tshammler A. Is the appearance of microcalcifications on mammography useful in predicting histological grade of malignancy in ductal cancer in situ. Br J Radiol 2000; 73: 938–44.
6. Hermann G, Keller RJ, Drossman S, Caravella BA, Tartter P, Panetta RA, Bleiweiss IJ. Mammographic pattern of microcalcifications in the preoperative diagnosis of comedo ductal carcinoma in situ: histopathologic correlation. Can Assoc Radiol J 1999; 50: 235–40.
7. Tan PH, Ho JTS, Ng EN, Chiang GSC, Low SC, Ng FC, Bay BH. Pathologic–radiologic correlations in screen-detected ductal carcinoma in situ of the breast: findings of the Singapore breast screening project. Int J Cancer 2000; 90: 231–6.
8. Tabar L, Gad A, Parsons WC, Neeland DB. Mammographic appearances of in situ carcinomas. In: Silverstein MJ, Ed. Ductal Carcinoma In

Situ of the Breast. Williams & Wilkins 1997, pp. 95–118.

9. Fisher ER, Dignam J, Tan-Chiu E, Costantino J, Fisher B, Paik S, Wolmark N. Pathologic findings from the National Surgical Adjuvant Breast Project (NSABP) 8-year update of Protocol B-17: intraductal carcinoma. Cancer 1999; 86: 429–38.

10. Bijker N, Peterse JL, Duchateau L et al. Risk factors for recurrence and metastasis after breast-conserving therapy for ductal carcinoma in situ: analysis of European Organization for Research and Treatment of Cancer Trial 10853. J Clin Oncol 2001; 19: 2263–71.

11. Bijker N, Peterse JL, Duchateau L et al. Histological type and marker expression of the primary tumour compared with its local recurrence after breast-conserving therapy for ductal carcinoma in situ. Br J Cancer 2001; 84: 539–44.

12. Solin LJ, Haffty B, Fourquet A et al. An international collaborative study: a 15-year experience. In: Silverstein MJ, Ed. Ductal Carcinoma In Situ of the Breast. Williams & Wilkins 1997, pp 385–90.

13. Holland R, Hendriks JH, Vebeek AL, Mravunac M, Schuurmans Stekhoven JH. Extent, distribution, and mammographic/histological correlations of breast ductal carcinoma in situ. Lancet 1990; 335: 519–22.

14. Rampaul RS, Valasiadou P, Pinder SE, Evans AJ, Wahedna Y, Wilson ARM, Ellis IO, Macmillan RD, Blamey RW. Wide local excision with 10-mm clearance without radiotherapy for DCIS. Eur J Cancer 2001: 37: 15.

15. Silverstein MJ, Lagios MD, Groshen S et al. The influence of margin width on local control of ductal carcinoma in situ of the breast. N Engl J Med 1999; 340: 1455–61.

16. Lamb PM, Perry NM, Vinnicombe SJ, Wells CA. Correlation between ultrasound characteristics, mammographic findings and histological grade in patients with invasive ductal carcinoma of the breast. Clin Radiol 2000; 55: 40–4.

17. Macmillan RD, Purushotham AD, Cordiner C, Dobson H, Mallon E, George WD. Predicting local recurrence by correlating preoperative mammographic findings with pathological risk factors in patients with breast cancer. Br J Radiol 1995; 68: 445–9.

18. Walls J, Knox F, Baildam AD, Asbury DL, Mansel RE, Bundred NJ. Can preoperative factors predict for residual malignancy after breast biopsy for invasive breast cancer? Ann R Coll Surg Engl 1996: 77: 248–51.

19. Kollias J, Gill PG, Beamond B, Rossi H, Langlois S, Vernon-Roberts E. Clinical and radiological predictors of complete excision in breast-conserving surgery for primary breast cancer. Aust NZ J Surg 1998; 68: 702–6.

20. Liljegren G, Lindgren A, Bergh J, Nordgren H, Tabar L, Holmberg L. Risk factors for local recurrence after conservative treatment in stage I breast cancer. Definition of a group not requiring radiotherapy. Ann Oncol 1997; 8: 235–41.

21. Faverly DR, Hendriks JH, Holland R. Breast carcinomas of limited extent: frequency, radiologic–pathologic characteristics, and surgical margin requirements. Cancer 2001; 91: 647–59.

22. Beron PJ, Horwitz EM, Martinez AA et al. Pathologic and mammographic findings predicting the adequacy of tumor excision before breast-conserving therapy. Am J Roentgenol 1996; 167: 1409–14.

23. Vicini FA, Recht A, Abner A et al. Recurrence in the breast following conservative surgery and radiation therapy for early-stage breast cancer. J Natl Cancer Inst 1992; 11: 33–39.

24. Healey EA, Osteen RT, Schnitt SJ, Gelman R, Stomper PC, Connolly JL, Harris JR. Can the clinical and mammographic findings at presentation predict the presence of an extensive intraductal component in early stage breast cancer? Intl J Radiat Oncol Biol Phys 1989; 17: 1217–21.

25. Tabar L, Chen HH, Duffy SW, Yen MF, Chiang CF, Dean PB, Smith RA. A novel method for prediction of long-term outcome of women with T1a, T1b, and 10–14 mm invasive breast cancers: a prospective study. Lancet 2000; 355: 429–33.

26. Brem RF, Behrndt VS, Sanow L, Gatewood OM. Atypical ductal hyperplasia: histologic underestimation of carcinoma in tissue harvested from impalpable breast lesions using 11-gauge stereotactically guided directional vacuum-assisted biopsy. Am J Roentgenol 1999; 172: 1405–7.

27. O'Hea BJ, Tornos C. Mild ductal atypia after large-core needle biopsy of the breast: is surgical excision always necessary? Surgery 2000; 128: 738–43.

28. Gadzala DE, Cederbom GJ, Bolton JS et al. Appropriate management of atypical ductal hyperplasia diagnosed by stereotactic core needle breast biopsy. Ann Surg Oncol 1997; 4: 283–6.

29. Moore MM, Hargett CW III, Hanks JB, Fajardo LL, Harvey JA, Frierson HF Jr, Slingluff CL Jr. Association of breast cancer with the finding of atypical ductal hyperplasia at core breast biopsy. Ann Surg 1997; 225: 726–31.

30. Adrales G, Turk P, Wallace T, Bird R, Norton HJ, Greene F. Is surgical excision necessary for atypical ductal hyperplasia of the breast diagnosed by Mammotome? Am J Surg 2000; 180: 313–15.

31. Luini A, Zurrida S, Paganelli G et al. Comparison of radio-guided excision with wire localisation of occult breast lesions. Br J Surg 1999; 86: 522–5.

32. Rampaul RS, Bagnall M, Burrell H, Wilson ARM, Vuyaic P, Pinder SE, Geraghty JG, Macmillan RD, Evans AJ. Prospective randomised study comparing radio-guided surgery (ROLL) to wire-guidance for occult breast lesion localisation. Eur J Cancer 2001: 37: 2–3.

9

High-frequency ultrasound

W. L. Teh

Introduction

The mainstay of detection of microcalcifications is mammography. As the typical size of microcalcifications ranges from 50 to 500 microns in size, mammography is well suited to the task of demonstrating the presence of breast microcalcifications. Using modern screen-film combinations, microcalcifications of 50 microns in size can be detected. The morphology of microcalcifications can be further characterised using magnification views. Magnification views enable the microcalcifications to be further analysed according to the degree of clustering, density, morphology and distribution as well as whether any other associated features such as the presence of any masses or distortions. Indeterminate and suspicious clusters of microcalcifications can then be localised and biopsied under stereotactic guidance in order to achieve a histological diagnosis. For ultrasound to be of clinical use in the diagnosis of microcalcifications, the efficacy in the detection, analysis, classification and guidance of biopsy procedures must be measured against that of conventional screen-film mammography. The ability to detect suspicious clustered microcalcification in breast screening is particularly important as it enables the detection of DCIS, which may be associated with small high histological grade invasive tumours[1].

Background

The early literature using automated whole breast water-path scanners in the early 1980s shows that palpable or mammographic masses containing calcifications appear as masses containing internal echoes or areas of acoustic attenuation.

Microcalcifications could not be positively identified. The limiting factor may be the low frequency (3.7–4 MHz) that is responsible for the poor lateral resolution of 2 mm[2,3].

However, microcalcifications larger than 0.5 mm could be differentiated as strong echogenic foci in hypoechoic masses. The main value was the ability to demonstrate masses that were associated with invasive carcinoma.

The introduction of higher frequency 7.5 MHz transducers with automatic scanners improved visualisation of microcalcifications; Jackson et al.[4] were able to detect microcalcifications sonographically in 57% of cases but only when associated with masses. The use of real-time 7.5 MHz transducers further improved detectability of microcalcifications as actual echogenic foci in hypoechoic areas[5]. These tend to appear larger than the actual pathological size and do not attenuate. Using 7.5–10 MHz real-time ultrasound equipment, ultrasound abnormalities corresponding to clustered microcalcifications can be identified in 59.6–76% cases with a specificity for malignancy of 82–93%[6–8]. There is, however, lower accuracy in the positive identification of benign microcalcifications. Not all malignant microcalcifications could be positively identified on ultrasound; this is usually due to the absence of a definite sonographic mass. There is also no clear distinction in whether the malignant lesions identified sonographically were invasive carcinoma, which were usually associated with a sonographic mass or pure in situ disease. Other investigators using similar equipment to localise impalpable lesions presenting solely as microcalcifications have not been able to achieve this level of detection[9–11].

The use of higher frequency ultrasound probes (HFUS) with operating frequencies above 7.5 MHz and claimed axial and lateral resolution of 0.1–0.5 mm improved the ability of detecting microcalcifications, and this appeared to be substantiated by investigators using 10 and 13 MHz transducers in the mid-1990s[12,13]. For instance, a 5–10 MHz broadband transducer with axial and lateral resolutions of 0.9 mm and 1.1 mm, respectively, is capable of detecting micro-calcifications greater than 0.6 mm in size[14]. This compares to the detection of microcalcifications of 0.15 mm in size, which can be identified using a 13 MHz transducer with an axial resolution of 0.118 mm. However, the results are mixed with sensitivities ranging from 52% (31/52 patients) to 88% (15/17 patients)[8,13,15]. The ability to visualise micro-calcifications is likely to be multifactorial, depending not only on the presence of any associated sonographic abnormalities but also on operator experience.

Technique and application

The use of a broadband width linear trans-ducer with a mid-frequency above 7.5 MHz improves the axial (defined by the pulse width) and lateral resolution (defined by echo beam width). Identification of the area of interest is best guided by the knowledge of the mammographic location; this is easiest if the true lateral and cranio-caudal projections are used. The conventional orthogonal scan-ning planes can be used initially. Scanning in the radial and anti-radial planes is particu-larly useful when there is a high suspicion of a ductal pathology where the mammograms suggest a ductal or segmental distribution with pleomorphic clustering of microcalcifi-cations.

More recently, there have also been attempts to improve detection of malignant disease associated with microcalcifications by using colour or power Doppler ultrasound. Malignant breast disease is associated with neoangiogenesis in invasive breast cancer and increased vascularity in high-grade DCIS[16–18]. In a recent study involving 44 patients, power Doppler vascularity associated with clustered microcalcifications was identified in 4/14 (28.6%) benign lesions and 12/30 (40%) malignant lesions[19]. The presence of focal power Doppler vascularity was instrumental in detecting focal small masses or distortions in eight cases, which in turn aided ultrasound core biopsy. In total, the combination of power Doppler and 13 MHz transducer enabled the visualisation of isolated clustered microcalci-fication in 93% of cases.

Where an ultrasound abnormality has been identified, it is essential that it be corre-lated with the mammographic appearance.

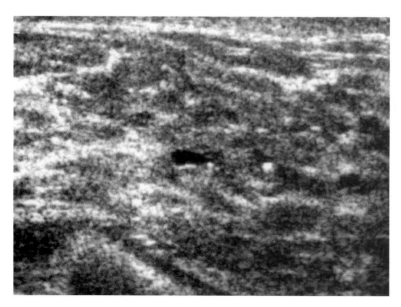

Fig. 10.1
Benign microcalcifications in stromal fibrosis manifest as echogenic foci in relatively hypoechoic breast tissue.

In the presence of suspicious clustered micro-calcifications, the presence of a mass or echo-poor attenuating area should be considered suspicious for malignant disease. A positive ultrasound correlate is amenable to percutaneous needle biopsy under ultrasound guidance. In the absence of a sonographic mass, the sonographic lesion may still be amenable to ultrasound-guided needle biopsy. In this situation, specimen radiography should be undertaken to ensure that representative microcalcification is obtained. The use of a large volume percutaneous sampling device such as the Mammotome™ is likely to improve the diagnostic yield where the sonographic appearance is subtle or manifest as hyper-echoic foci in the absence of a mass.

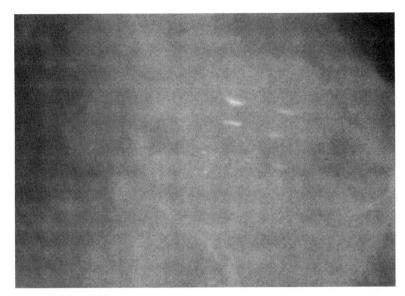

Fig. 10. 2
Lateral magnification view showing typical "tea-cupping" of milk of calcium in microcysts.

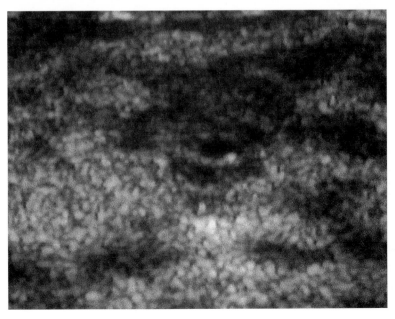

Fig. 10.3
Ultrasound image depicting microcysts with milk of calcium layering within the cysts.

10

Ultrasound appearances of benign microcalcifications

Benign calcifications can be difficult to identify as many of these occur in fibro-glandular tissue where there is lack of contrast required to distinguish the echogenic foci within the echogenic tissue. The presence of stromal flecks of hyperechoic foci representing stromal calcifications can sometimes be clearly identified (Fig. 10.1). Small microcysts containing "milk of calcium" as well as areas of focal fibrocystic change containing microcalcifications are

Table 10.1 Detectability of clustered microcalcifications in prospective studies with histological correlation

Authors	Transducer frequency	Benign	Malignant in situ	Malignant invasive
Yang et al 1997[14]	5–10 MHz linear broadband	–	0 (0/6)	Invasive only 100% (36/36) DCIS and invasive 52.4% (22/42)
Ranieri et al 1997[8]	10 MHz annular	33.3% (7/21)	33.3% (3/9)	95.4% (21/22)
Cleverley et al 1997[13]	10/13 MHz linear	87.5% (7/8)	87.8% (7/8)	–
Gufler et al 2000[24]	7.5 MHz linear	59.2% (16/27)	100% (9/9)	100% (11/11) 8/11 invasive with in situ
Moon et al 2000[21]	5–10 and 5–12 MHz linear	22.6% (14/62)	76.7% (23/30)	100% (8/8)
Teh 2000[19]	13 MHz linear and power Doppler	85.7% (12/14)	85.7% (6/7)	100% (10/10 invasive with in situ)

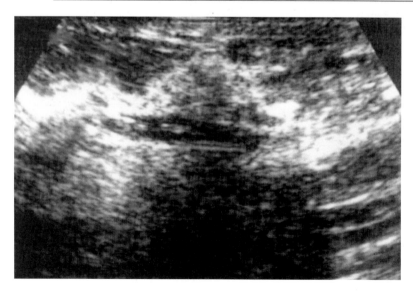

Fig. 10.4
A 13 MHz annular array image showing a dilated duct containing echogenic foci. There is associated parenchymal hypoechogenicity. The surgical diagnosis is high-grade DCIS.

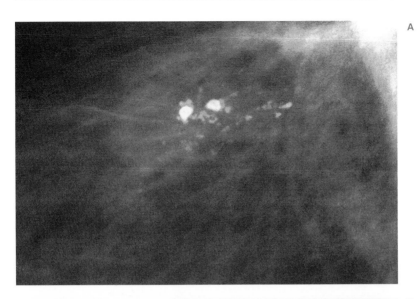

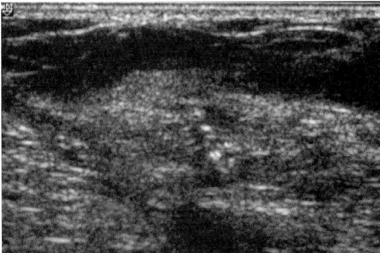

Fig. 10.5
(A) Mammogram showing segmental distribution of clustered malignant microcalcifications. (B) Ultrasound images confirm the presence of strongly echogenic foci. An ultrasound-guided core biopsy and subsequent surgical excision confirms comedo DCIS.

other positive benign findings (Figs 10.2 and 10.3). Fibroadenomas containing flecks of attenuating coarser calcifications are also usually visible due to the presence of an associated hypoechoic mass. Nevertheless the definitive identification of benign microcalcification is comparatively lower from that of malignant disease and ranges from 33.5% to 85.7% in prospective studies where histological correlation is available (Table 10.1).

Ultrasound appearances of malignant-type microcalcifications

Malignant lesions are usually more readily identified even in the absence of a mammographic mass. The detectability varies depending on whether the microcalcifications are associated with DCIS or whether there is any associated invasive carcinoma. Comparative studies generally show detection of pure DCIS to be superior to that of benign disease but inferior to that in which invasive disease is also present (Table 10.1). Morphological features described in DCIS include the presence of dilated ducts containing flecks of microcalcifications (Fig. 10.4)[20]. There may be associated sonographic parenchymal changes or hypoechoic lesions.

Adjacent strongly echogenic foci representing microcalcifications are also generally seen (Fig. 10.5). Masses or irregular attenuating areas may also be present particularly with high-grade or comedo DCIS (Fig. 10.6)[20–22]. These have the appearances of the typical spiculated or irregular masses or non-strongly attenuating lesions or distortions. In

A

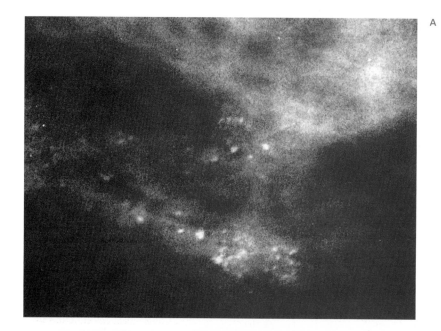

B

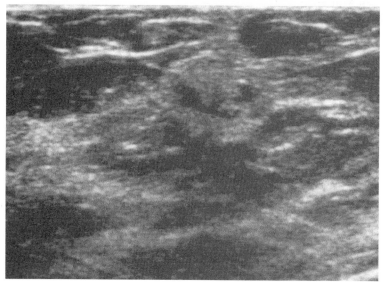

Fig. 10.6
(A) Magnification view of clustered casting microcalcifications.
(B) Ultrasound of the area demonstrates the presence of several irregular masses with associated parenchymal changes. A fleck of strongly echogenic focus is seen within the irregular mass. Ultrasound core biopsy confirms high-grade DCIS.

some cases, masses are not seen but secondary signs of surrounding parenchymal abnormality (such as increased echogenicity of the intramammary fat) may be present. Where invasive carcinoma is present, the positive identification of a sonographic abnormality approaches that of 100%. These tend be irregular, ill-defined masses. The ability to visualise a sonographic abnormality is particularly high where the mammogram shows a suspicious (e.g. pleomorphic or typically casting or comedo pattern) appearance or where there is clustering of more than 10 mm in extent. The increased detection rate of malignant calcifications using ultrasound has been successfully exploited by investigators as a means of performing ultrasound-guided needle biopsy or localisations[8,13,19,21–23].

Summary

The use of high-frequency ultrasound can be used to detect mammographic microcalcifications. The ability to reliably detect benign microcalcifications remains low. Nevertheless, clustered suspicious microcalcifications demonstrated on mammography can be visualised using ultrasound, particularly where associated with malignancy. Malignant clustered microcalcifications of suspicious appearances, particularly if extensive, can be detected as either masses or focally dilated ducts. The use of power Doppler may also improve the detection of invasive foci of disease.

References

1. Evans AJ, Pinder SE, Snead DR, Wilson AR, Ellis IO, Elston CW. The detection of ductal carcinoma in situ at mammographic screening enables the diagnosis of small, grade 3 invasive tumours. Br J Cancer 1997; 75: 542–4.
2. Kopans DB, Meyer JE, Steinbock RT. Breast cancer: the appearance as delineated by whole breast water-path ultrasound scanning. J Clin Ultrasound 1982; 10: 313–22.
3. Lambie RW, Hodgden D, Herman EM, Kopperman M. Sonomammographic manifestations of mammographically detectable breast microcalcifications. J Ultrasound Med 1983; 2: 509–14.
4. Jackson VP, Kelly-Fry E, Rothschild PA, Holden RW, Clark SA. Automated breast sonography using a 7.5-MHz PVDF transducer: preliminary clinical evaluation. Work in progress. Radiology 1986; 159: 679–84.
5. Kasumi F. Can microcalcifications located within breast carcinomas be detected by ultrasound imaging? Ultrasound Med Biol 1988; 14 (Suppl 1): 175–82.
6. Leucht WJ, Leucht D, Kiesel L. Sonographic demonstration and evaluation of microcalcifications in the breast. Breast Dis 1992; 5: 105–23.
7. Kasumi F, Sakuma H. Identification of microcalcifications in breast cancers by ultrasound. In: Madjar H, Teubner J, Hackeloer B-J, Eds. Breast Ultrasound Update. Basel: Karger, 1994, pp. 154–67.
8. Ranieri E, D'Andrea MR, D'Alessio A et al. Ultrasound in the detection of breast cancer associated with isolated clustered microcalcifications, mammographically identified. Anticancer Res 1997; 17: 2831–5.
9. Pamilo M, Soiva M, Anttinen I, Roiha M, Suramo I. Ultrasonography of breast lesions detected in mammography screening. Acta Radiol 1991; 32: 220–5.
10. Potterton AJ, Peakman DJ, Young JR. Ultrasound demonstration of small breast cancers detected by mammographic screening. Clin Radiol 1994; 49: 808–13.
11. Rissanen TJ, Makarainen HP, Apaja-Sarkkinen MA, Lindholm EL. Mammography and ultrasound in the diagnosis of contralateral breast cancer. Acta Radiol 1995; 36: 358–66.
12. Kenzel PP, Hadijuana J, Schoenegg W, Minguillon C, Hosten N, Felix R. Can the high-resolution 13-MHz ultrasonography facilitate the preoperative localization and marking of microcalcification clusters? Rofo 1996; 6: 551–6.
13. Cleverley JR, Jackson AR, Bateman AC. Preoperative localization of breast microcalcification using high-frequency ultrasound. Clin Radiol 1997; 52: 924–6.
14. Yang WT, Suen M, Ahuja A, Metreweli C. In vivo demonstration of microcalcification in breast cancer using high resolution ultrasound. Br J Radiol 1997; 70: 685–690.
15. Cilotti A, Bagnolesi P, Moretti M et al. Comparison of the diagnostic performance of high-frequency ultrasound as a first- or second-line diagnostic tool in non-palpable lesions of the breast. Eur Radiol 1997; 7: 1240–4.
16. Engels K, Fox SB, Whitehouse RM, Gatter KC, Harris AL. Distinct angiogenic patterns are

associated with high-grade in situ ductal carcinomas of the breast. J Pathol 1997; 181: 207–12.

17. Lee AH, Happerfield LC, Bobrow LG, Millis RR. Angiogenesis and inflammation in ductal carcinoma in situ of the breast. J Pathol 1997; 181: 200–6.

18. Guidi AJ, Fischer L, Harris JR, Schnitt SJ. Microvessel density and distribution in ductal carcinoma in situ of the breast. J Natl Cancer Inst 1994; 86: 614–19.

19. Teh WL, Wilson AR, Evans AJ, Burrell H, Pinder SE, Ellis IO. Ultrasound-guided core biopsy of suspicious mammographic calcifications using high frequency and power Doppler ultrasound. Clin Radiol 2000; 55: 390–4.

20. Hashimoto BE, Kramer DJ, Picozzi VJ. High detection rate of breast ductal carcinoma in situ calcifications on mammographically directed high-resolution sonography. J Ultrasound Med 2001; 20: 501–8.

21. Moon WK, Im JG, Koh YH, Noh DY, Park IA. US of mammographically detected clustered microcalcifications. Radiology 2000; 217: 849–54.

22. Schoonjans JM, Brem RF. Sonographic appearance of ductal carcinoma in situ diagnosed with ultrasonographically guided large-core needle biopsy: correlation with mammographic and pathologic findings. J Ultrasound Med 2000; 19: 449–57.

23. Rickard MT. Ultrasound of malignant breast microcalcifications: role in evaluation and guided procedures. Australas Radiol 1996; 40: 26–31.

24. Gufler H, Buitrago-Tellez CH, Madjar H et al. Ultrasound demonstration of mammographically detected microcalcifications. Acta Radiol 2000; 41: 217–21.

11

Computer-aided detection of mammographic calcifications

Sue Astley

Introduction

Most mammograms are acquired on X-ray film. However, in recent years, digital X-ray acquisition systems have been developed, in which the information in the image is represented directly as a matrix of numbers (pixels). Although digital images may be printed on film for conventional viewing, they are more usually displayed and viewed on screen. Advances in digital acquisition and display technology, coupled with the flexibility offered by digital imaging, have made the prospect of routine digital mammography more realistic, although resolution is still an issue, particularly for screening applications where the early detection of microcalcifications is important.

The use of digital mammograms offers a number of significant advantages. First, the images are readily amenable to manipulation by performing mathematical operations on the matrix of numbers. Such processing can facilitate viewing; for example, by adjusting the contrast or brightness, or by using knowledge of the imaging physics to compensate for degradation[1]. Specific image features can be made more – or less – conspicuous to aid the detection of abnormalities; for instance, linear structures might be enhanced to improve visualisation of architectural distortion, or suppressed to aid detection of masses. Quantitative information can also be extracted to enable classification of detected abnormalities for diagnostic purposes, or measurement for monitoring response to treatment. Images of the left and right breast, or films taken on different occasions, may be registered to facilitate comparison. A further advantage of using digital images is that they can be rapidly transmitted to other sites, and multiple copies may be made available without loss of image quality. Digital images can be easily annotated without detriment to the original data; multiple annotations can thus be acquired for teaching and research pur-

poses. Intelligent software has been developed to provide access to digital image databases, not only on the basis of finding several examples of a given pathology, but to enable searches for images which share particular properties. This is useful both for teaching and for diagnostic purposes.

One of the most exciting prospects is that of using a computer to automatically detect groups of pixels corresponding to clinically significant abnormalities[2]. Research in this area has been active for the last 25 years, with an increase in interest and particularly rapid progress during the last 10 years. Most of the algorithms to date have been developed and tested using digitised film images. Detection of mammographic abnormalities is a challenging problem both for human and computer, due to the sometimes ill-defined and subtle nature of abnormal signs, the complexity and variability of the underlying mammographic structure and the similarity of normal and abnormal image features. This is compounded, in the screening context, by the infrequency of clinically significant abnormalities and by the requirement for efficiency. The most successful results to date have been for the detection of microcalcification clusters; although these may pose a problem of perception for the human observer, they have a well-defined range of appearance and are dissimilar to the parenchymal background. Current algorithms are capable of detecting a very high percentage of microcalcification clusters with a low false positive rate. There has also been good progress on the detection of spiculated masses, by virtue of the fact that a combination of radiating linear stucture and a bright central region is not typical of the underlying background, but the results so far are less impressive than those for microcalcification detection. Some signs of abnormality, in particular asymmetry and distortion, are even more difficult to detect. For these signs, there is less agreement between human observers

11

11

about what constitutes a significant degree of abnormality, or merely a variation of normal appearance. Further algorithms have been developed to analyse detected abnormalities with a view to improving the benign biopsy rate and providing additional diagnostic information. Again, the most successful attempts at this are directed at the classification of calcification.

Computer-aided mammography

The aim of much of the early research into abnormality detection was to replace the human film reader by a fully automatic computerised system. However, in order to do this, the computer must be able reliably to detect all manifestations of mammographic abnormality with both a very high sensitivity and an acceptably low false positive rate. Clearly, at present, it is not feasible to use a machine even as an automatic second reader; the only type of abnormality for which detection performance approaches the levels attained by experienced human film readers is microcalcification.

Another potential model for computer-aided mammography is prescreening, in which the screening films are sorted by the computer into two groups: those that are unequivocally normal and those that may contain an abnormality. The radiologist would then look only at those films classified as potentially abnormal, reviewing just a small number of the normal group for quality control purposes. Provided a sufficient proportion of the films are correctly identified as being unequivocally normal, this model would focus the radiologist on the more difficult and abnormal films, making better use of their skills. Technically, this requires algorithms that can either reliably detect normal images or that can detect all

manifestations of abnormality with great sensitivity – but not necessarily with high specificity. The detection of normality is an area in which research is active; a starting point is the classification of mammograms according to their glandular background, as this has been shown to be related to risk[3,4]. Detection of abnormalities is easier in fatty breasts for both human and machine, and a significant proportion of women in the screening age group have predominantly fatty breasts, so it may be that a combined approach could enable prescreening. Current computer-aided detection systems are not designed for prescreening; the full range of abnormalities is not usually targeted, and too large a proportion of mammograms are flagged with suspicious regions to make prescreening cost-effective.

There is, however, a way in which computer-based detection algorithms can be used to aid the process of detecting mammographic abnormalities without having a full suite of algorithms, and without the requirement that the algorithms must be almost perfectly sensitive. There is now evidence that computer-based prompting can improve human detection performance. The idea of prompting is to attract the reader's attention to regions of the original image which may be abnormal. First, the computer uses algorithms to detect potential abnormalities, and their locations are presented to the human film reader as prompts, which are usually small symbols or outlines of suspicious regions superimposed on a low resolution version of the mammogram. The human reader, having first viewed the original image unaided, consults the prompt image and reviews the original image accordingly. Some of the prompts may correspond to genuine abnormalities which the human reader either failed to see in their initial search of the mammogram, or to abnormalities which they saw but dismissed as being insignificant.

This approach is known as computer-aided detection (CAD) and, with the advent of commercial CAD systems, we are beginning to understand the parameters which make prompting effective. Clearly, the algorithms need to be sensitive, and to detect not only the more obvious abnormalities but also subtle signs that would otherwise be missed or dismissed by human readers. However, there is also evidence that too many false prompts reduce the benefits offered by the technology[5]. This could happen by a number of different mechanisms. For example, false prompts could distract the human reader, drawing attention away from regions containing genuine abnormalities. If there are a large number of false prompts, the radiologist's confidence in the significance of prompts might also be reduced, causing him to routinely ignore prompting information. Most commercial CAD systems are centred around a highly sensitive microcalcification detection algorithm, along with at least one other algorithm (usually to detect masses). As all the prompts are presented on a single prompt image, the response of the human reader is complex, even though microcalcification and mass prompts are distinct. There is published evidence that CAD system algorithms are capable of detecting very early cancers; researchers have looked at the previous screening films of women with interval cancers, and found that a number of these had prompts in the right place[6]. Despite this, there is as yet no evidence that a commercial CAD system can improve the performance of human readers in the context of the National Health Service Breast Screening Programme.

Microcalcification detection

Microcalcifications are sometimes difficult for the human film reader to detect because of their small size and low contrast, particularly if there are only a few particles, and if these are superimposed on dense glandular tissue. However, of all the signs of abnormality found on mammograms, microcalcifications are the easiest for computers to deal with. Unlike small ill-defined masses, which may superficially resemble normal glandular tissue, microcalcifications have properties that differ significantly from those of normal background structures. Their small size is, in this respect, an advantage, as is their relatively high attenuation coefficient. The computer can be trained to detect small, bright, regions with well-defined edges. Most algorithms make an initial attempt at detection, followed up by a more specific analysis to reduce the number of false positive responses. The small size of microcalcification particles necessitates the use of very high-resolution digital images in which many pixels are used to represent each square millimetre of the mammogram. The more pixels in the image, the longer it takes to process, so the initial detection stage is used to reduce the number of pixels at which detailed further analysis will be applied.

False signals may be generated by overlapping narrow linear structures, or artifacts such as screen-film "shot" noise, but these can generally be excluded by further analysis[7]. The analysis phase focuses both on the properties of individual candidate particles – shape, size and brightness – and also on the distribution of candidate particles within the image. One of the most powerful tools for reducing the false positive rate of detection algorithms is the application of clustering criteria; generally, a detection is only registered (and prompted) if a number of individual bright regions are found within a limited area. In other words, prompts are only placed where clusters of calcifications are found.

A more difficult problem is distinguishing between calcifications that would be dismissed as insignificant by experienced radiologists and those it is imperative to detect and prompt. Unless highly accurate characterisation algorithms are available, it is probably safer to prompt all clusters and leave the decision as to whether any further action should be taken to the radiologist. A loss of confidence in microcalcification prompts could result if some clusters are prompted and some are not.

There have been many published papers describing methods for detecting microcalcifications in digital mammograms, but it is difficult to compare their efficacy because few have been applied to the same sets of data. The majority of researchers work with local clinicians and have relied on these clinicians to provide images considered to be representative examples. This is a highly subjective approach, as there are considerable differences in opinion as to what constitutes a representative data set. Some examples are much less conspicuous than others, and whilst a number of researchers have attempted to compensate for this by classifying lesions according to subtlety, it is difficult to avoid bias. In addition, differences in data arise because some data sets are based on screening mammograms and others on symptomatic cases, and because of differences in screening practice.

The problem of subjectivity can be avoided by using large samples (either randomly selected or consecutive) taken from screening data. In this way, examples with multiple abnormality types and common artifacts will be naturally included. The performance on very early cancers can be measured using suitably reviewed previous screening films from interval cancer cases, and normal data should be taken from the previous screening films of women who have had a subsequent normal screening examination.

Further difficulties in evaluating algorithms arise because of the nature of the ground truth against which the computer's performance is compared. As the majority of computer-based detection methods are applied to screening and symptomatic mammograms, it is extremely difficult to get accurate pathological evidence of the location of abnormalities – especially for microcalcifications. We must rely on annotations provided by experts, and once again the problem of subjectivity arises. In the main, only the boundaries of calcification clusters are marked, rather than individual particles, as annotation of individual particles is extremely time-consuming and difficult, generally requiring access to both the digital image and the original film. To facilitate comparison of methods, public databases of digitised mammograms have been made available[7].

The majority of attempts to automatically detect microcalcification clusters in digital mammograms have directly exploited the most obvious properties of the particles: their small size, their increased brightness compared to their backgrounds and their relatively sharp edges. There exist many generic computer vision techniques which can be used to detect small bright blobs or edges in images, and researchers have applied several of these to mammograms. One class of techniques which has been investigated for the detection of microcalcifications by a number of researchers is mathematical morphology[9-11]. The mammogram may be considered as a surface, raised according to brightness, with small peaks corresponding to microcalcifications, and larger ones corresponding to other structures. Morphological operations such as erosion and dilation modify the surface according to a predefined structuring element, and combinations of modified surfaces can be used to enhance structures of particular sizes and shapes. Unfortunately, such simple techniques also detect any noise peaks of similar size and shape present in the images, and poor classification of image pixels into calcification versus non-calcification results. These results improve when clustering rules are applied, and sensitivities of approximately 95% with about 0.5 false clusters per image have been reported[11]. Morphology may also be helpful in identifying suspicious regions, based on an examination of the distribution of detected peak sizes in normal and abnormal tissue[12].

There are similarities between the morphological approaches and that developed by Chan and colleagues[13]. Their method involves subtracting an image in which the microcalcifications have been suppressed from one in which they have been enhanced by means of a matched filter. Following subtraction, there are several stages of post-processing involving extraction of potential microcalcifications and subsequent feature analysis. More recently, methods based on neural networks have been used to reduce the number of false positive clusters. A sensitivity of 93.3% (measured on a 'per case' basis) with 0.7 false clusters per image has been obtained[14].

An alternative approach is to attempt to detect the edges of calcification particles by amplifying gradient information in the images. However, there are a large number of edges naturally present in mammograms, all of which will be enhanced, and the subsequent task of determining which edges correspond to microcalcifications is complex. Various combinations of edge and peak detection have been investigated, but none has achieved sufficient sensitivity and specificity to be clinically useful.

A more sophisticated method was devised by Karssemeijer, who devised a statistical preprocessing algorithm for noise estimation and equalisation which was found to significantly improve results[15]. Each pixel is assigned one of four labels: background, microcalcification, line/edge, or film emulsion error. The detection method, based on the use of Bayesian techniques and a Markov random field model to describe spatial relationships between pixel labels, involves iteratively updating the labels to maximise their probability. The method uses both contrast and edge information. A cluster was defined as at least two detections in an area enclosed by an empty region half a centimetre wide. Results, plotted on FROC curves, showed a sensitivity of more than 90% with slightly less than one false detection per image on a set of 40 mammograms.

Finally, commercial CAD systems are now under evaluation both in the UK and abroad. The detection performance of some of the algorithms is impressive; the ImageChecker system from R2 Technology can currently detect over 86% of all abnormalities in NHSBSP films. However, the microcalcification detection algorithm far outshines the system's mass detection capabilities, and whilst the ImageChecker produces very few false microcalcification prompts (approximately one in every four cases), on average there is at least one false mass prompt per case. Despite this, the system is still the most specific commercial system available.

Conclusions

Just a few examples of computer-based methods for detecting microcalcifications are discussed here; many more have been described in the literature, and still more are under development. The most successful methods can detect 98% of microcalcification clusters, but in most cases, their false positive rates are still too high to enable effective prompting. A rate of 0.5 false prompts per image may sound good, but for a four-film mammogram this rate corresponds to an average of two false prompts per case, and the vast majority of cases will have at least one false prompt.

Many of the false prompts for microcalcification detection algorithms correspond to clusters or image features an experienced film reader would simply dismiss, and it may be that work on characterisation and classification of microcalcification clusters

11

will pave the way for more detailed analysis of candidate clusters. Characterisation research has, to date, focused both on the properties of individual particles (for example, size, shape and density) and on the properties of clusters (overall cluster shape and distribution of particles). Some of these features – especially cluster shape – are very difficult to deal with because of the nature of the imaging process. Three-dimensional cluster shapes are projected into a two-dimensional image; even if the effects of breast compression are small, robust characterisation of the projected shapes is difficult, especially for clusters of only a few particles.

In summary, the detection of microcalcification clusters is the most successful application of computer-based detection in mammography. This is due to the differences between microcalcifications – notably size and attenuation coefficient – and their background. A great deal of research effort has been directed at their detection, with the result that most clusters can be detected automatically, although false positive detections due to artifacts and other background structures may occur. For automated detection to be a useful tool, the false positive rate must be reduced even further and, if they are to be incorporated into a CAD system, the false prompt rates of algorithms for other abnormalities must also be reduced significantly.

References

1. Highnam R, Brady JM. Mammographic Image Analysis. Dordrecht: Kluwer Academic, 1998.
2. Boggis CRM, Astley SM. Computer-assisted mammographic imaging. Breast Cancer Res 2000; 2: 392–4.
3. Byng JW, Critten JP, Boyd NF et al. Analysis of digitized mammograms for the prediction of breast cancer risk. In: Doi K, Giger ML, Nishikawa RM, Schmidt RA, Eds. Proceedings of the Third International Workshop on Digital Mammography. Amsterdam: Elsevier, 1996, pp. 185–90.
4. Wolfe JN. Risk for breast cancer development determined by mammographic parenchymal pattern. Cancer 1976; 37: 2486–92.
5. Astley SM, Zwiggelaar R, Wolstenholme C, Davies K, Parr TC, Taylor CJ. Prompting in mammography: how good must prompt generators be? In: Karssemeijer N, Thijssen M, Hendriks J, van Erning L, Eds. Digital Mammography. Dordrecht: Kluwer Academic Publishers, 1998, pp. 347–54.
6. Warren Burhenne LJ, Wood SA, D'Orsi CJ et al. Potential contribution of computer-aided detection to the sensitivity of screening mammography. Radiology 2000; 215: 554–62.
7. Poissonier M, Brady M. Noise equalization, film-screen artifacts, and density representation. In: Yaffe MJ, Ed. Proceedings of the Fifth International Workshop on Digital Mammography. Wisconsin: Medical Physics Publishing, 2001, pp. 605–11.
8. Heath M, Bowyer K, Kopans D, Moore R, Kegelmeyer P. The digital database for screening mammography. In: Yaffe MJ, Ed. Proceedings of the Fifth International Workshop on Digital Mammography. Wisconsin: Medical Physics Publishing, 2001, pp. 212–18.
9. Astley S, Taylor C. Detection of microcalcifications in mammograms. In: Proceedings of the First British Machine Vision Conference, 1990.
10. Rick A, Muller S, Bothorol S, Grimaud M. Quantitative modeling of microcalcification detection in digital mammography. In: Proceedings of the Medical Image Computing and Computer-Assisted Intervention, 1999, pp. 32–41.
11. Hagihara Y, Kobatake H, Nawano S, Takeo H. Accurate detection of microcalcifications on mammograms by improvement of morphological processing. In: Yaffe MJ, Ed. Proceedings of the Fifth International Workshop on Digital Mammography. Wisconsin: Medical Physics Publishing, 2001, pp. 193–7.
12. Bruynooghe M. High resolution granulometric analysis for early detection of small microcalcification clusters in X-ray mammograms. In: Yaffe MJ, Ed. Proceedings of the Fifth International Workshop on Digital Mammography. Wisconsin: Medical Physics Publishing, 2001, pp. 154–60.
13. Chan H-P, Doi K, Galhotra S, Vyborny C, MacMahon H, Jokich P. Image feature analysis and computer-aided diagnosis in digital radiography. (I) Automated detection of microcalcifications in mammography. Med Physics 1987; 14: 538–48.
14. Gurcan MN, Chan H-P, Sahiner B, Hadjiiski L, Petrick N, Helvie MA 2002 Optimal Neural Network Architecture Selection: Improvement in the Computerized Detection of Microcalcifications. Academic Radiology 9: 420–29.
15. Karssemeijer N. Adaptive noise equalisation and recognition of microcalcification clusters in mammograms. Intl J Pattern Recognition Artif Intelligence 1993; 7: 1357–76.

Chapter

12

MRI detection of DCIS

Fiona J. Gilbert

Introduction

Initial experience with MRI suggested that breast examination was not very useful as there is overlap of T1 relaxation times of breast parenchymal tissue, benign lesions and malignant disease. Following the introduction of intravenous gadolinium-based contrast medium it was found that dynamic contrast-enhanced breast MRI was very sensitive to the detection of malignancy[1]. There have been a number of publications indicating sensitivities of between 88 and 100% but with variable lower specificity (Table 12.1).

The rapid leakage of contrast into the extravascular, extracellular space in cancers is responsible for the change in signal. The local paramagnetic effects on T1-weighted images shortening the relaxation time, resulting in increased signal, allows detection of abnormalities, particularly if the high signal from the adjacent fat is suppressed by using either a fat-suppression technique or image subtraction.

Lesion morphology, enhancement patterns and signal change over time are used to differentiate benign disease from malignant tissue. Features suggesting malignancy are an enhancing mass with irregular or spicu-lated margins[2]. In a series of 56 malignant lesions, 50 had these features, giving a positive predictive value for malignancy of 89%[3]. Benign masses have smooth or lobulated borders and have non-enhancing internal septations[2]. Lesions with these characteristics and non-enhancing lobulated masses were found to be benign in 52 cases, with a negative predictive value for malignancy of 100%[4]. Smooth masses most often represented fibrocystic change, and lobulated masses with non-enhancing internal septations were most likely to be fibroadenomas. DCIS is the most common histological correlate of ductal enhancement, with a positive predictive value of 40%. Enhancement in one region of the breast (regional enhancement) is usually due to fibrocystic change or malignancy (PPV 42%). Of these malignancies, half are DCIS and half are DCIS with an invasive component[4].

Enhancement patterns are also thought to be important in improving benign/malignant differentiation. In order to evaluate lesion enhancement, images need to be acquired every minute sequentially before and after injection of contrast for up to 5–8 minutes. Large data sets are produced and the limitation on the number of sequences

Table 12.1 Overall sensitivity and specificity of MRI

Author	Year	No. of patients	No. of cancers	Benign lesions	Sensitivity (%)	Specificity (%)
Heywang et al.[26]	1989	150	71	27	98	65
Kaiser & Zeitler[27]	1989	191	58	31	100	97
Harms et al.[24]	1993	30	47	27	94	37
Oellinger et al.[28]	1993	33	25	16	88	80
Gilles et al.[29]	1994	143	64	79	95	53
Boetes et al.[30]	1994	83	65	22	95	86
Orel et al.[18]	1995	176	72	112	92	88
Bone et al.[9]	1996	231	155	95	93	73
Nunes et al.[31]	1997	94	46	48	96	79
Kuhl et al.[32]	2001	192	15		100	

12

acquired dynamically is the capacity of the software to process the data. The T1 signal change can be plotted over time to demonstrate the initial rate of contrast enhancement, the peak signal and subsequent signal change.

Strong, early enhancement with a relative signal increase of over 140% and a peak of enhancement before 3 minutes is highly suggestive of malignancy together with early washout, i.e. a signal decrease of more than 10% following maximum enhancement. Focal, irregular and non-homogeneous enhancement or enhancement that follows a ductal pattern is suspicious. Rim or centripetal enhancement, i.e. enhancement that starts at the periphery and progresses towards the centre of an abnormality, is highly suggestive of malignancy. However, it is becoming increasingly clear that both enhancement characteristics and lesion morphology are required to separate benign and malignant lesions[2].

MRI was initially not thought to be useful in the detection of DCIS. With increasing asymptomatic mammographic screening, the proportion of DCIS cases had increased from 5% of all breast cancers to 15–20% of all detected breast cancers and 25–30% of all clinically occult cancers detected by mammography[5]. Due to this increased detection of DCIS, recent breast MRI series have included larger numbers of DCIS and radiologists have also examined the utility of breast MRI to improve the diagnosis in mammographically detected microcalcification.

MRI sensitivity and specificity in DCIS

Most of the published breast MRI series have been consecutive patients with either clinical or mammographic abnormalities. DCIS has been found together with invasive ductal carcinoma and the sensitivity and specificity for MRI for DCIS have been calculated as a sub-analysis[4,6–11]. MRI is performed for a variety of reasons, usually suspicious mammographic features, palpable lump on clinical examination or newly diagnosed breast cancer. DCIS tends to represent only a small proportion of the patients in the series. The cases are identified retrospectively and then the characteristic features of DCIS are analysed. In almost all of the series, the MRI examinations are read with the knowledge and availability of the mammograms, with few series reporting the MRI examination blind. Sensitivity of MRI for the detection of DCIS in these series varies between 77% and 100%, the specificity varying between 28% and 100% (Table 12.2).

The value of MRI as a problem-solving tool in patients with mammographic microcalcification has been examined in two series. Westerhoff et al.[12] examined 63 consecutive patients with suspicious isolated clustered microcalcification to assess the additional value of MRI in relation to surgical management. In this cohort, 33 patients had DCIS, five patients invasive ductal cancer and 25 patients had benign disease. The overall accuracy of MRI was 56%, with 45% sensitivity and 72% specificity. The sensitivity for detection of DCIS was 67%. In this series, the MRI did not detect any additional disease that had not been identified on mammography and did not alter surgical management[12].

A large, prospective two-centre study included 172 women with isolated, clustered, suspicious microcalcification. All were destined for excision biopsy and examined with dynamic contrast-enhanced MRI. Eight malignant lesions were found, of which 58 were in situ cancers and 22 invasive carcinoma. The remaining 92 women had benign lesions. The overall sensitivity was 95% with MRI detecting early enhancement in 56 of 58 cases of in situ disease[6]. However, while a high sensitivity was achieved, the authors concluded that specificity was poor, limiting

Table 12.2 MRI detection of DCIS

Author	Year	No. of patients	No. of patients with DCIS	Sensitivity	Specificity
Gilles et al.[6]	1996	172	58	95%	51%
Bone et al.[9]	1996	231	17	82%	73%
Soderstrom et al.[8]	1996	22	22	100%	–
Orel et al.[7]	1997	330	13 pure	77%	–
Westerhof et al.[12]	1998	63	33	67%	72%
Kuhl et al.[16]	1998	33	33	100%	–
Nunes et al.[4]	1999	192	11	90%	–
Hiramatsu et al.[33]	1999	21	17	15/17	100%
Amano et al.[11]	2000	58	26	19/26	–
Satake et al.[13]	2000	46	15	91%	–
Viewheg et al.[15]	2000	71	50	96%	28%

12

the value of MRI in distinguishing benign and malignant mammographic microcalcification.

Overall, the sensitivity of breast MRI in detection of DCIS is lower than for invasive disease. The reasons for this are complex and are discussed below. Sensitivity is improved if the mammogram is available to direct attention to areas of suspicious microcalcification. The specificity is variable and similar to invasive disease.

Morphology of DCIS

DCIS typically displays clumped or linear enhancement with a ductal distribution. Less commonly, DCIS can show a spiculated appearance or even ring enhancement, although infiltrating invasive disease is more likely to cause a spiculated appearance[8]. Ill-defined or diffuse enhancement in a segmental distribution tends to be the most common finding. Satake, in a study designed to compare ultrasound detection of intraductal spread with mammography and MRI, found three morphological patterns – linear, regional and segmental enhancement, with segmental and linear being the most common correlate of DCIS[13]. Nunes, in attempting to correlate lesion appearance with histological findings for a breast MRI interpretation model, found 11 cases of DCIS in a series of 192 patients. MRI detected 10 of these 11 cases, four had ductal enhancement (ductal is linear and branching), four regional enhancement (where regional is defined as diffuse, ill-defined pattern), one irregular mass and one spiculated mass[4]. Linear, spotty enhancement, an area of linear enhancement, an enhancing area or mass without distortion of the surrounding tissue and a well-circumscribed mass have all been found on MRI and reported in a series of 10 cases of DCIS[14]. The spectrum of DCIS morphology is well demonstrated in Viewheg's series of 50 patients. Of the 48 lesions showing enhancement, the commonest appearance was of an ill-defined area of enhancement followed by a well-defined area, the remaining lesions demonstrating a ductal pattern (eight cases) and a diffuse area of enhancement in five cases[15]. Segmentally extended enhancement defined as vague, faint and diffuse enhancement forming a

12

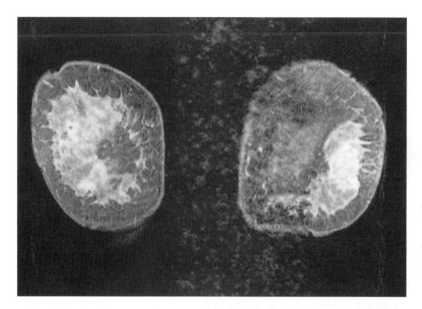

Fig. 12.1 A
Postcontrast T1-weighted image with 3-cm invasive ductal carcinoma showing heterogeneous enhancement and an irregular margin in the lower outer quadrant of the left breast.

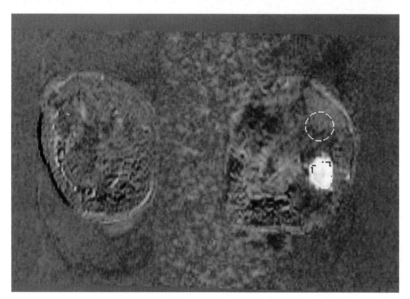

Fig. 12.1 B
Subtraction of pre- and postcontrast T1-weighted image improves conspicuity of abnormal enhancing area caused by invasive ductal carcinoma. Regions of interest drawn round the enhancing tumour and also round adjacent fat. The subtracted image results in fat suppression.

segmental "cone" shape was found in four pure DCIS lesions, and 10 predominantly DCIS cases with multiple focal masses confined to one quadrant were found in three DCIS cases. No enhancement was found in seven cases of DCIS associated with invasive cancer[11].

Fibrocystic enhancement patterns are most likely to be confused with DCIS. Benign proliferative changes are seen as fine stippled enhancement[8]. Fibrocystic and proliferative change appears as ill-defined irregular segment or region of enhancement which is a common appearance of DCIS. In summary,

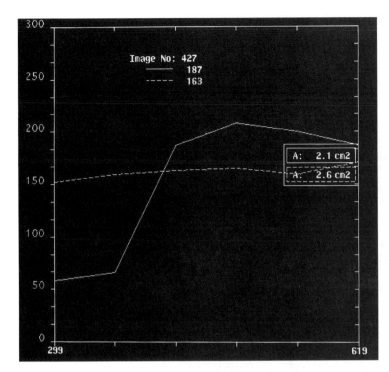

Fig. 12.1 C
Time signal enhancement curve demonstrates rapid rise in enhancement peak reached within 2 minutes and more than 10% wash out immediately following peak enhancement. The enhancement curve is typical of invasive carcinoma (type III curve). The background fat signal shown by the dotted line shows a slow steady rise in signal by approximately 10%.

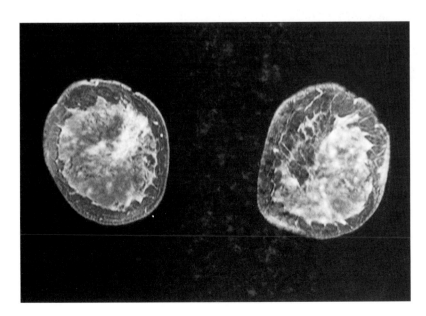

Fig. 12.2 A
Wedge-shaped area of enhancement seen at the 2 o'clock position of the right breast on postcontrast T1-weighted images.

12

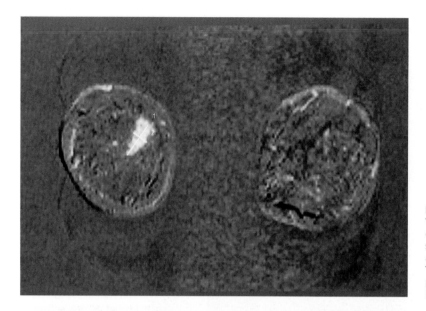

Fig. 12.2 B
Wedge-shaped segmental area of enhancement on fat-suppressed images created by a subtraction of precontrast T1-weighted images from postcontrast T1-weighted image.

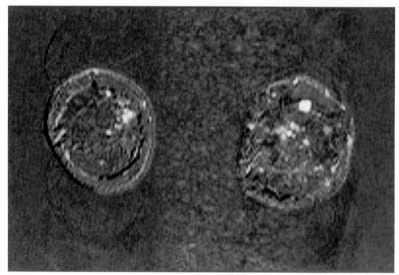

Fig. 12.2 C
Adjacent slice with a rather linear ductal pattern at the 2 o'clock position of the right breast. On the left breast there is an irregular lobulated lesion at the 12 o'clock position which was a further 1.2 cm area of invasive ductal cancer. The segmental area of enhancement is due to DCIS.

any focal area with diffuse ill-defined enhancement should be considered suspicious and investigated further. Enhancement following a linear, branching or ductal pattern should be considered suspicious of DCIS. Rarely, a focal or spiculated mass can be due to DCIS and this should be remembered when reporting this type of abnormality.

Enhancement rate

DCIS enhancement rates can be very variable with some lesions enhancing rapidly and some slowly. Classically, invasive malignancy enhances early and reaches a peak within 3 minutes of injection time. Contrast injection in the antecubital vein to breast enhancement is thought to take approxi-

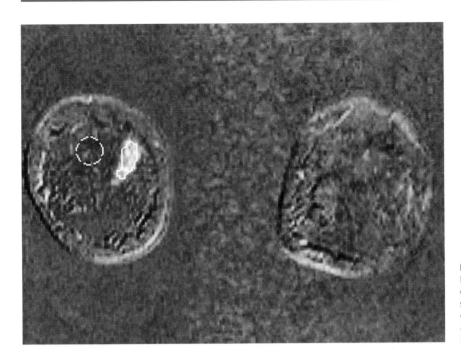

Fig. 12.2 D
Region of interest
drawn around
segmental area of
enhancement and
adjacent area of
background fat.

12

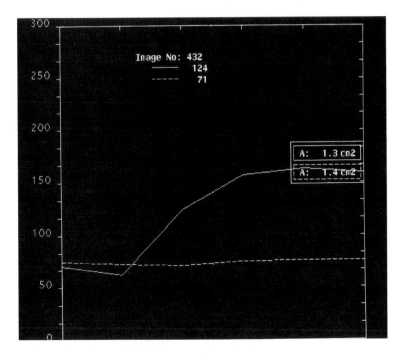

Fig. 12.2 E
Graph demonstrates signal change
over time. Images acquired at
1-minute intervals. Continuous line
shows slow continuous
enhancement over time with no
wash out. This type II curve is
commonly found with DCIS as in this
case. Again, background fat shows
little change in signal over time.

mately 46 seconds, although this will vary with heart rate and rapidity of the bolus injection. Hiramatsu et al. found that DCIS tended to be slowly enhancing in 10 cases of pure DCIS[14]. In a larger series of 50 cases of pure DCIS, enhancement was delayed in 65% of lesions[15]. The majority of cases showed strong enhancement, with 16 showing indeterminate enhancement and five low enhancement, and in only two cases was enhancement absent[15]. Kuhl et al.'s[16] series of 33 patients showed fast enhancement in 49%, intermediate enhancement in 30% and delayed in 21% with all patients with DCIS showing some enhancement. The time–signal intensity curves showed type I, steadily increasing, in 73%, with type II, early rise and plateau, in 18% and type III, peak with washout, in 9%, whereas invasive disease typically shows the reverse, i.e. 8%, 27% and 65%, respectively[16]. Similarly, in Viehweg's series, only 4% of DCIS showed the malignant washout pattern[15].

In the differentiation of DCIS from benign disease it is unhelpful to use enhancement rates, as the rapid enhancement characteristic of invasive disease is often not present in DCIS. The enhancement patterns of benign proliferative change tend to overlap those of DCIS with slow continuous enhancement. This can result in DCIS being overlooked. On finding slow diffuse enhancement, it is important to review the mammograms to search for evidence of DCIS. Most authors advocate interpretation of breast MRI only in conjunction with the mammograms. If the morphological changes are consistent with DCIS then a biopsy should be considered. It is important to retain a high index of suspicion when diffuse enhancement patterns are even. Timing of the examination is important as during the second half of the menstrual cycle the normal breast parenchyma can show marked enhancement. Imaging is recommended between days 6 and 16 of menstrual cycle to reduce over-investigation

of parenchymal changes[17]. HRT can cause similar effects and it is suggested stopping HRT 4 weeks prior to examination to reduce the number of enhancing normal areas of breast tissue.

Relationship between DCIS tumour grading and MR enhancement

There does not appear to be a relationship between the grading of DCIS and the rate of contrast enhancement, or even whether the DCIS displays any signal change[14]. There is no significant difference between the rate of enhancement according to grade, the presence or absence of necrosis or microinvasion. Although 76% of comedo DCIS showed focal early enhancement, compared to only 50% of non-comedo DCIS, no relationship between contrast enhancement and tumour grade has been found[12]. Again, in Orel's series of 19 patients with DCIS (13 pure DCIS and six DCIS with separate foci of invasive disease), there was no correlation between grade of tumour and enhancement. MRI detected seven of nine cases with comedo high grade, three out of six non-comedo intermediate grade and three out of three non-comedo low grade[18]. Viehweg found ductal enhancement more common in comedo-type DCIS (29%) compared to non-comedo (12%). Comedo DCIS was more likely to have early enhancement (50%) compared to non-comedo (29%), although none of these were shown to be statistically significant[15].

Lack of enhancement is the reason for most false negative cases in the literature. False negative cases of both comedo and non-comedo type DCIS have been reported[18]. Stomper et al. reported three false negative cases, including a 4-cm area of comedo DCIS with 1 mm of microinvasion, and a second 6-cm area of comedo[19]. The one false negative case in Sataki's series was comedo DCIS in the sub-areolar area[13]. The retro-areolar area is notoriously difficult to assess on MRI as well as mammographically. A 0.6-cm focus of DCIS did not enhance and was the cause of the one negative case in a series of 11 patients[4].

It is important to be aware that not all cases of DCIS enhance. As MRI is sometimes used as a problem-solving tool to exclude malignancy and, clearly, DCIS cannot be excluded using dynamic contrast-enhanced MRI as the negative predictive value is not as high for DCIS as it is for invasive disease.

Can MRI accurately demonstrate extent of DCIS?

The classical mammographic features of DCIS are irregular, linear or branching micro-calcifications with or without an associated ill-defined soft-tissue mass with, rarely, an ill-defined soft-tissue mass being the only finding. Mammography can underestimate the extent of disease, and this is a particular problem if DCIS is part of multifocal or multicentric pathology. The extent of DCIS demonstrated on MRI has been shown to correlate reasonably well with histological assessment[3,8,12]. Westerhof, in his series of 63 patients, found no additional disease on MRI or at histological examination compared to mammography[8]. Soderstrom et al., using the fat-suppressed RODEO technique, found the MRI estimation of disease extent concordant with pathology in 22 cases, the only exception being one case of pure DCIS where MRI overestimated disease extent – the clumping pattern was found which correlated with DCIS, fibrocystic change and sclerosing adenosis. In the same series, mammography enabled accurate prediction of disease extent in 14 of 19 (74%) patients[8].

While Gilles et al. found a significant correlation between the size of DCIS and histopathological analysis ($r = 0.85$, $P =$ 0.0085), they found that there were some differences in the correlation depending on the type of enhancement pattern. When focal enhancement was seen, there was a good correlation with size at histological examination, in 20 out of 26 patients, but in the remaining six MRI underestimated the extent of disease. Where there was early diffuse enhancement, in only two out of eight patients was there accurate histological correlation and, in the remaining patients, MRI overestimated the extent of DCIS. This was thought to be due to adjacent proliferative disease (four patients) or non-proliferative fibrocystic change[3].

MRI has demonstrated mammographically occult DCIS. In one series of 15 cases of DCIS found on MRI, five of the cases were not detected by mammography[20]. Similarly, in the series reported by Orel of 19 DCIS cases detected on MRI, seven were mammographically occult and six of these had multifocal disease (three in the same quadrant and three in a separate quadrant)[7]. In a series of 33 consecutive DCIS cases, 20 were mammographically occult[21].

While MRI can demonstrate additional disease, the false negative cases mentioned in the previous section show that it is not as accurate as histological examination. On balance, MRI is probably as good as mammography in demonstrating the extent of DCIS.

Does type of sequence used influence MRI detection of DCIS

Most breast MRI studies have been performed on high field strength systems (1.0–1.5 T). These produce good signal-to-noise ratios, allow spectrally selected fat suppression and increase the T1 relaxation times of tissues increasing the signal difference between native and contrast-enhanced tissue.

Dedicated phased array breast coils allow

12

12

excellent spatial resolution and, with modern hardware and software, allow good temporal resolution. These requirements are necessary for the detection of small foci of DCIS. Fat suppression is necessary to increase lesion conspicuity as subtraction techniques are hampered by patient movement which can obscure small abnormalities. Bilateral breast imaging is recommended due to high incidence of bilateral disease (3–6%)[22], either in the axial or coronal plane.

A variety of strategies have been employed to improve both detection of small cancers and DCIS. This has mainly been by improving spatial resolution and signal-to-noise ratio. Use of contrast is necessary to detect malignant lesions. The dose used is normally 0.1 ml/kg, although some protocols have recommended a double dose to improve lesion conspicuity[23]. Ideally, voxels less than 3 mm should be achieved by using slice thickness < 3 mm, with as small a rectangular field of view as possible to reduce volume averaging. T1-weighted sequence precontrast with postcontrast sequences repeated up to 5–8 times are recommended with each sequence lasting fewer than 60–90 seconds.

The detection of small foci of DCIS appears to be improved by the use of fat-suppressed three-dimensional volume spoiled gradient echo sequences (SPGR)[7]. Both Harms and Soderstrom have claimed that three-dimensional rotating delivery of excitation off resonance (3D RODEO) sequence, which is fat-suppressed, has improved contrast and spatial resolution. In 22 cases of DCIS, the true extent of disease was demonstrated in 21 of 22 cases[8]. Harms et al. demonstrated the value of this sequence initially and demonstrated DCIS in all seven cases[24]. It is thought that the magnetisation transfer contrast inherent in the RODEO sequence improves the contrast-to-noise ratio between cancer and ductal tissue, which reduces the effects of volume averag-

ing between DCIS and normal parenchyma. Also it is claimed that the microcalcification can be detected directly on MRI as it produces magnetic susceptibility artefacts. However, the susceptibility effects does not help distinguish between benign and malignant disease[8].

New techniques have been introduced in an attempt to improve the temporal resolution of breast imaging. Dynamic spiral MRI achieves improved temporal resolution but at a cost of lowering spatial resolution. The 7–10 mm section thickness leads to greater volume averaging, resulting in decrease in lesion detection. The technique therefore needs to be combined with high spatial resolution conventional fat-suppressed images. With spiral MRI, the susceptibility artefacts are greater due to the longer readout time and the lack of magnetisation transfer suppression of muscle and normal fibroglandular tissue. In six cases of DCIS there was variable contrast enhancement. The technique was very useful for utilising the exchange rate constant to differentiate benign from invasive disease but it was not helpful in separating DCIS from benign disease[10].

Polarity-altered spectral and spatial selective acquisition (PASTA) technique for fat suppression has been used with three-dimensional fast spin echo sequences. PASTA uses narrow band spectral selective 90° pulse to eliminate fat, and a reverse polarity 180° pulse to avoid contamination of fat signals from other sections. Ando reported a series of 49 women imaged using this technique, in which there were seven DCIS cases[25]. The method detects tumour vascularity directly instead of evaluating pattern of enhancement and this could be used as a surrogate marker of malignancy. In the initial patients in the series, two-dimensional fast spin echo sequences were used with three to six slices 6-mm thick, but latterly a three-dimensional fast spin echo sequence was used in the sagittal plane. Maximum intensity projections are created and peritumoural, intratumoural and marginal vascularity is documented. Intratumour and marginal vascularity were significantly more common in invasive disease than in DCIS but DCIS could not be reliably differentiated from benign disease.

Conclusion

The sensitivity of MRI to detect DCIS is lower than for invasive cancer, likely due to the variable angiogenesis found with DCIS. The most specific patterns are linear, clumped, regional and segmental enhancement but more commonly a diffuse, ill-defined pattern is seen. Signal change following contrast tends to be less than invasive disease but greater than benign, proliferative changes. The enhancement rate can be rapid but more commonly is slow, continuing to rise or plateau, with washout rarely seen. There is no relationship to grade of in situ disease. High resolution imaging is required to detect DCIS together with a high index of suspicion when dealing with ill-defined, diffusely enhancing areas.

References

1. Heywang-Kobrunner S, Hahn D, Schmid H, Krischke I, Eiermann W, Bassermann R, Lissner J. MR imaging of the breast using gadolinium DTPA. J Comput Assist Tomogr 1986; 10: 199–204.
2. Orel S. MR imaging of the breast. Radiol Clin N Am 2000; 38: 899–913.
3. Gilles R, Zafrani B, Guinebretiere J et al. Ductal carcinoma in situ: MR imaging – histopathological correlation. Radiology 1995; 196: 415–19.
4. Nunes L, Schnall M, Orel S, Hochman M, Langlotz C, Reynolds C, Torosian M. Correlation of lesion appearance and histologic findings for the nodes of a breast MR imaging interpretation model. Radiographics 1999; 19: 79–92.
5. Stomper P, Margolin F. Ductal carcinoma in situ: the mammographer's perspective. Am J Roentgenol 1994; 162: 585–91.
6. Gilles R, Meunier M, Lucidarme O et al. Clustered breast microcalcification: evaluation by dynamic contrast-enhanced subtraction MRI. J Comput Assist Tomogr 1996; 20: 9–14.
7. Orel S, Mendonca M, Reynolds C, Schnall M, Solin L, Sullivan D. MR imaging of ductal carcinoma in situ. Radiology 1997; 202: 413–20.
8. Soderstrom C, Harms S, Copit D et al. Three-dimensional RODEO breast MR imaging of lesions containing ductal carcinoma in situ. Radiology 1996; 201: 427–32.
9. Bone B, Aspelin P, Bronge L, Isberg B, Perbeck L, Veress B. Sensitivity and specificity of MR mammography with histopathological correlation in 250 breasts. Acta Radiol 1996; 37: 208–13.
10. Daniel B, Yen Y, Glover G et al. Breast disease: dynamic spiral MR imaging. Radiology 1998; 209: 499–509.
11. Amano G, Ohuci N, Ishibashi T, Ishida T, Amari M, Satomi S. Correlation of three-dimensional magnetic resonance imaging with precise histopathological map concerning carcinoma extension in the breast. Breast Cancer Res Treat 2000; 60: 43–55.
12. Westerhof J, Fischer U, Moritz J, Oestmann J. MR imaging of mammographically detected clustered microcalcifications: is there any value? Radiology 1998; 207: 675–81.
13. Satake H, Shimamoto K, Sawaki A et al. Role of ultrasonography in the detection of intraductal spread of breast cancer: correlation with pathologic findings, mammography and MR imaging. Eur Radiol 2000; 10: 1726–32.
14. Hiramatsu H, Ikeda T, Mukai M, Masamura S, Kikuchi K, Hiramatsu K. MRI of ductal carcinoma in situ of the breast: patterns of findings and evaluation of disease extent. Nippon Igaku Hoshasen Gakkai Sasshi 2000; 60: 205–9.
15. Viehweg P, Lampe D, Buchmann J, Heywang-Kobrunner S. In situ and minimally invasive breast cancer: morphologic and kinetic features on contrast-enhanced MR imaging. Magn Reson Materials Physics Biol Med 2000; 11: 129–37.
16. Kuhl C, Mielcarek P, Leutner C, Schild H. Diagnostic criteria of ductal carcinoma in-situ (DCIS) in dynamic contrast-enhanced breast MRI: comparison with invasive breast cancer (IBC) and benign lesions. Proc Intl Soc Mag Reson Med 1998; 2: 931
17. Brown J, Buckley D, Coulthard A et al. Magnetic resonance imaging screening in women at genetic risk of breast cancer: imaging and analysis protocol for the UK multicentre study. UK MRI Breast Screening Study Advisory Group. Magn Reson Imag 2000; 18: 765–76.
18. Orel S, Schnall M, Powell C, Hochman M, Solin L, Fowble B, Torosian M, Rosato E. Staging of suspected breast cancer: effect of MR imaging and MR-guided biopsy. Radiology 1995; 196: 115–22.

12

19. Stomper P, Herman S, Klippenstein D et al. Suspect breast lesions: findings at dynamic gadolinium-enhanced MR imaging correlated with mammographic and pathologic features. Radiology 1995; 197: 387–95.

20. Heywang-Kobrunner S. Contrast-enhanced MRI of the breast. Invest Radiol 1994; 29: 94–104.

21. Abraham D, Jones R, Jones S et al. Evaluation of neoadjuvant chemotherapeutic response of locally advanced breast cancer by magnetic resonance imaging. Cancer 1996; 78: 91–100.

22. Fischer U, Kopka L, Grabbe E. Breast carcinoma: effect of preoperative contrast-enhanced MR imaging before re-excisional biopsy. Radiology 1999; 213: 881–8.

23. Brown J, Coulthard A, Dixon A et al. Protocol for a national multi-centre study of magnetic resonance imaging screening in women at genetic risk of breast cancer. Breast 2000; 9: 78–82.

24. Harms S, Flamig D, Hesley K et al. MR imaging of the breast with rotating delivery of excitation off resonance: clinical experience with pathologic correlation. Radiology 1993; 187: 493–501.

25. Ando Y, Fukatsu H, Ishiguchi T, Ishigaki T, Endo T, Miyazaki M. Diagnostic utility of tumor vascularity on magnetic resonance imaging of the breast. Magn Reson Imag 2000; 18: 807–13.

26. Heywang S, Wolf A, Pruss E, Hilbertz T, Eiermann W, Permanetter W. MR imaging of the breast with Gd-DTPA: use and limitations. Radiology 1989; 171: 95–103.

27. Kaiser W, Zeitler E. MR imaging of the breast: fast imaging sequences with and without Gd-DTPA. Radiology 1989; 170: 681–6.

28. Oellinger H, Heins S, Sander B. Gd-DTPA-enhanced MR breast imaging: the most sensitive method for multicentric carcinomas of the female breast. Eur Radiol 1993; 3: 223–6.

29. Gilles R, Guinebietier J, Lucidarme O et al. Non-palpable breast tumours: diagnosis with contrast-enhanced subtraction dynamic MR imaging. Radiology 1994; 191: 625–31.

30. Boetes C, Barentsz J, Mus R et al. MR characterisation of suspicious breast lesions with a gadolinium-enhanced TurboFLASH subtraction technique. Radiology 1994; 193: 777–81.

31. Nunes L, Schnall M, Orel SG, Hochman M, Langlotz C, Reynolds C, Torosian M. Breast MR imaging: interpretation model. Radiology 1997; 202: 833–41.

32. Kuhl C, Schmutzler R, Leutner C et al. Breast MR imaging screening in 192 women proved or suspected to be carriers of a breast cancer susceptibility gene: preliminary results. Radiology 2000; 215: 267–79.

33. Hiramatsu H, Enomoto K, Ikeda T et al. Three-dimensional helical CT for treatment planning of breast cancer. Radiat Med 1999; 17: 35–40.

12

The nature of breast tissue calcifications

K. D. Rogers and R. A. Lewis

A crystallographic perspective

The formation of crystalline and semi-crystalline materials occurs extensively within biological tissues due to natural biological processes, disease, drug therapies and implants. However, detailed crystallographic study of these organic and inorganic materials has generally been very limited, with perhaps the exception of bone. Traditionally, crystallographers determine and examine details of the regular atomic distributions associated with crystalline solids by exploiting diffraction phenomena. Measurements of intensity distributions from diffraction experiments are utilised to "solve" crystal structures. Further information associated with structural disorder (e.g. crystallite size and "strain" and atomic substitutions), is also available from diffraction data. Such ultrastructural characteristics have marked effects upon macroscopic properties and behaviour of materials such as reactivity and hardness. Crystallographic descriptions of materials' microstructures can provide information about formation mechanisms, formation environments and an indication of how the crystals will interact with their environment.

Frequently, crystalline materials associated with biological tissues are calcific minerals. These have been exploited diagnostically when located in pathological tissues such as the brain[1], thorax[2], liver[3], arteries[4], joints[5] and retina[6]. The most common biological mineral, found in a wide range of crystalline forms and body locations, is based upon the prototype structure of calcium hydroxyapatite $[Ca_{10}(PO_4)_6(OH)_2]$. In vivo it occurs with extensive ionic substitution, e.g. carbonate ions replacing the indigenous hydroxy or phosphate ions and, hence, it shall be referred to as b-HAP within this chapter. This material forms the bulk of bone and teeth. As expected after many years of in vivo development, b-HAP has ideal properties to behave as both an ion store and mechanical composite matrix. However, this apatite is also the most common form of dystrophic and metastatic mineral.

Other than bone and teeth, the most well known and studied human mineralisation is associated with the urinary system (crystalluria and urolithiasis), although the crystalline constituents of uroliths are not exclusively mineral in nature[7]. Uroliths have been extensively structurally characterised and found to consist of a wide range of crystalline materials that most often combine to form elegant, laminar architectural macrostructures.

Currently, an important part of initial breast cancer diagnosis is based upon the mammographic appearance of radio-opaque deposits commonly thought to be calcification. Such mammographically recognised calcification has been used, for some time, to indicate high-risk areas within breast tissues[8,9] and increased specificity may be gained from magnification of the images[10]. Indeed it has even been suggested that medial calcific sclerosis of breast arteries may also be diagnostic[11] and that the shape of the crystallites on mammograms can be instructive[12]. The prognostic value of calcification has also been examined and a significantly greater number (twice as many) of lymph nodes appear to be involved with tumours of patients with calcification[13]. This has suggested the possibility of calcium deposition being related to tumour cell metastasis.

Despite extensive diagnostic use made of these deposits (albeit with a relatively low specificity[14]), the detail of their chemical and structural composition has not been fully determined. Thus, the clinical significance of breast tissue calcifications as diagnostic indicators of tumour type and stage is far from being fully explored. Further, there is little evidence correlating the type of calcification to its mammographic appearance, e.g. the linear and granular distributions that have

13

been correlated to tumour subtype[15]. Also any relationship of calcific nature to histological classifications, such as that by Maria Foschini[16], has not been established. However, several studies have suggested that the type of calcification formed may act as a marker for malignancy and that simply the presence of calcification may be of biological significance; 5- and 20-year survival of patients with calcifications has been found to be significantly less than those without[17,18].

Currently, there are several contradictory and limited studies examining the diagnostic ability of the chemical nature of calcifications. Undoubtedly there is significant experimental confounding within and between these studies due to differences in sampling methods, specimen preparation/storage and analysis techniques. Crystallographic characterisation of these calcifications would certainly go some way to resolve many of these issues.

The aim of this chapter is to review the crystallographic data related to breast tissue calcifications and examine the implications and value of this information for (a) breast cancer diagnosis and (b) understanding the natural history of the disease. This review is, for the most part, observational but placed within an appropriate context. The processes and language associated with crystallography and diffraction are also introduced. Much of the initial background is presented in relation to b-HAP as this undoubtedly forms the majority mineral of breast tissue deposits.

Crystallographic structures of biogenic calcifications

The term "crystalline" is used to indicate the presence of long-range atomic order within a material. Within highly crystalline materials, such as silicon wafers used by the semiconductor industry, the regular arrangement of atomic units can persist over several centimetres and crystallographic investigations can be performed using single crystals. A more common material form, "polycrystalline", occurs when the crystal size (typically 0.1–100 µm) is many times smaller than the interrogating X-ray probe and many, randomly oriented, crystallites are present within the sample. Thus, although a high degree of atomic order exists within each crystallite, intercrystallite orientational order is absent. However, in some solid materials, the atomic order persists only over a single molecule (e.g. glasses) and such materials are referred to as "amorphous". This should not be confused with the frequent use of this term to describe the visual and mammographic appearance of breast tissue deposits; crystalline precipitates often form with an ill-defined visual morphology. Between the single crystal and amorphous extremes are intermediate states including "nanocrystalline" materials in which the crystallite size is only a few nanometers. In fact, bone mineral may be considered such a material and its extensive ultrastructural disorder (typical of all b-HAP) described by a "paracrystalline" model[19].

Biological calcifications are typically treated as polycrystalline, although it has been asserted that in vivo precipitation of amorphous calcium phosphate is a precursor stage in the formation of b-HAP.

Diffraction data (upon which crystallographic characterisation is based) from single crystal and polycrystalline forms are significantly different in nature and in the information that they can provide. For example, single crystal studies tend to provide relatively accurate and precise atomic position and vibrational data, whereas data from polycrystalline experiments, although possibly not as precise, may also provide crystallite morphology and other microstructural information. In particular, the "phase" (see following paragraph) of a material is routinely identified from polycrystalline data.

Conventionally, three-dimensional, atomic distributions in crystalline materials are reduced to a description of (a) the morphology of the molecular repeating unit or motif, known as the "unit cell" and defined by "lattice parameters", and (b) the atomic species and atom positions (or "sites") within a single unit cell. These concepts are illustrated, with reference to calcium hydroxyapatite, in Figure 13.1. Different crystalline materials are distinguished by differences in unit cell morphology and/or cell contents. Unique atomic distributions and cell morphologies are identified as "phases". Thus calcium hydroxyapatite, calcium oxalate monohydrate (COM) and calcium oxalate dihydrate (COD) are unique crystalline phases. However, within each crystalline phase, subtle differences in stoichiometry (e.g. the fraction of atomic sites occupied and atomic substitutions) and lattice parameters frequently exist. This is certainly the case for b-HAP that is almost exclusively found with hexagonal unit cell morphology – a phase

form of hydroxyapatite that is only stabilised by the inclusion of impurity atoms[20].

Usually, changes to unit cell contents effect the lattice parameters.* For example, in the range of biological interest, carbonate substitution for the PO_4 ions of calcium hydroxyapatite causes a contraction of the a-axis by 6.2×10^{-4} nm/wt% and an expansion of the c-axis by 2.3×10^{-4} nm/wt%[21]. Other ionic substitution effects in hydroxyapatite are indicated in Table 13.1. Similar effects are also observed when the hydration state of a material is changed, for example in calcium oxalates. Thus, accurate determination of lattice parameters can provide information on the precise nature of the material. However, an inherent difficulty of employing lattice parameters for interpretation of b-HAP stoichiometry, is the confounding effect of multiple heteroionic substitutions that often must occur for charge balance, e.g. when CO_3^{2-} is substituted for PO_4^{3-} in calcium hydroxyapatite, then a substitution of Na^+ for Ca^{2+} or loss of Ca is often observed[20]. Heteroionic substitutions in b-HAP are extensive. For example, a detailed study[22] of an enamel apatite determined its stoichiometry to be,

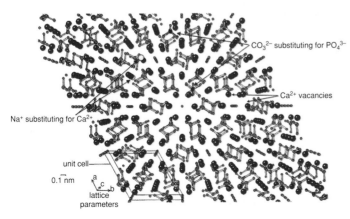

CO_3^{2-} substituting for PO_4^{3-}

Ca^{2+} vacancies

Na^+ substituting for Ca^{2+}

unit cell

0.1 nm

a

c b

lattice parameters

Fig. 13.1
Perspective view of HAP crystallographic structure as seen along the c-axis (along the O-H channels).

* It should be realised that much of the crystallographic data concerning hydroxyapatite is derived from the synthetic preparations of the mineral. Interpretation of structural data corresponding to b-HAP is derived from these synthetic studies.

Table 13.1 Qualitative description of lattice parameter changes in HAP resulting from ionic substitutions

Ion	Substitution	Lattice parameter changes
CO_3^{2-}	PO_4^{3-}	$a^1 c^2$
CO_3^{2-}	OH^-	$a^2 c^1$
F^-	OH^-	$a^1 c^3$
Cl^-	OH^-	$a^2 c^1$
Sr^{2+}	Ca^{2+}	$a^2 c^2$
Mg^{2+}	Ca^{2+}	$a^2 c^1$
Mn^{2+}	Ca^{2+}	$a^1 c^1$
Cd^{2+}	Ca^{2+}	$a^1 c^1$
Na^+	Ca^{2+}	$a^3 c^3$
Pb^{2+}	Ca^{2+}	$a^2 c^2$

[1,2] indicates an increase and decrease respectively,
[3] indicates no measurable change.

$$(Ca_{3.89}Na_{0.09}Mg_{0.02})_I(Ca_{5.59}Na_{0.13}Mg_{0.03})_{II}(PO_4)_{5.5}(CO_3)_{0.5}(OH)_{1.78}$$

(the I & II subscripts referring to different Ca sites within the unit cell).

Small changes to stoichiometry and crystallite microstructure often have a significant impact upon crystallite–environment interactions. For example, performance critical parameters of b-HAP crystallites within bone include their morphology and amount of carbonate substitution. Morphology is important for enzyme interactions, as these are specific to particular growth surfaces of hydroxyapatite[23]. Increased carbonate substitution has been shown to enhance significantly the reactivity and dissolution of synthetic hydroxyapatite in vitro[24]. Further, the inflammatory properties of crystallites within tissues have been shown to depend critically upon the chemical and microstructural characteristics (e.g. specific surface area) of the crystals[25]. The ability of HAP crystals to lyse cell membranes has a similar dependence[26].

The formation conditions associated with calcifications within breast tissues are important to assess; the extracellular environment in which crystallites form significantly affects both the unit cell contents and crystallite morphology. Thus, crystallographic detail of calcifications may be exploited to indicate local, dynamic changes in tissue physiology and/or metabolism, i.e. disease onset. In vitro studies have shown that changes to the morphology of growing crystallites occur in response to changes in environmental pH[27]. An early study[28] indicated a correlation between the nature of the calcifications formed and breast tissue pH. The pH is significantly higher within breast ducts than surrounding tissues and b-HAP direct precipitation requires an alkaline environment. Further, calcification morphogenesis may indicate if direct precipitation or phase transformation (for example from amorphous calcium phosphate) is occurring. Also crystallite morphology is influenced by preferential adsorption of proteins. In particular, HAP has a high affinity for protein adsorption but this is often associated with particular crystal faces. For example, bone acidic proteins have been shown to adsorb preferentially upon faces normal to the crystallite c-axis where calcium ions present a regular arrangement[23]. A consequence of this is preferential growth along the c-axis.

It is highly likely that the histopathological appearance of breast calcifications is directly influenced by the precise nature of mineral. For example, the granular and laminar calcifications of DCIS characterised by Foschini et al.[16] are clearly indicative of different crystallite growth environments and growth processes. Thus the crystallites' crystallographic features will inevitably be different. Although not specific to breast tissues, a comprehensive review of biological crystal formation in pathological tissues is provided by Daculsi et al.[29].

Characterisation of calcifications

When considering the microscopic and ultrastructural characterisation of biological tissues, it is important to appreciate the precise nature of information generated by various analytical methods. Traditionally, histopathological examination of tissues does not warrant the use of techniques that provide high specificity for crystalline phase. Stains such as Von Kossa and alizarin red, frequently used in the examination of breast tissues, are able to indicate high calcium concentrations and even provide a degree of phase differentiation through the use of further stains such as silver nitrate/rubeanic acid and H&E safranin. However, specificity is low and it has been suggested that traditional histopathological techniques can alter the hydration states of materials. Further, specimen storage methods may have a significant influence upon the inorganic tissue deposits[30]. The optical appearance of calcifications is certainly not phase-specific and, even using polarising microscopy, it can be misleading, for example when birefringency is thought specific for COD[12]. A critical evaluation of the use of polarising microscopy for

breast tissue calcification has recently been provided by the mineralogist Jill Pasteris, who concluded that there was significant misapplication of technique and misleading mineral identification within pathology literature[31].

Scanning electron microscopy (SEM) is an increasingly common and versatile analysis tool that can be applied to histopathological slides with little specimen preparation. However, in its usual imaging mode it suffers from the same specificity limitations as optical microscopy although it has significantly greater sensitivity. It has been recently shown[32] that SEM may detect calcifications missed by histopathology and, thus, it is highly likely that the frequency of calcification within breast and other tissues is significantly greater than currently reported. SEM studies tend to report crystalline deposits as a range of forms, from large aggregates to very small, fine needles. This clearly indicates differences in formation mechanisms and/or environments.

Most electron microscopes are modified to accommodate detectors that measure X-rays produced from the interactions between probe electrons and atoms within the sample. The energies of these X-rays are characteristic of the atoms within the specimens and thus this technique (known as electron beam microprobe, EBM, or X-ray microanalysis) provides information concerning the atomic species within tissues. It is occasionally, and unfortunately, confused with X-ray diffraction[33]. Although EBM is not easily quantifiable, it has been previously applied to breast tissue calcifications[34] where Ca/P ratios ranged from 1.5 to 1.7. Often it is mistakenly suggested that the technique is specific for phase; for example, calcium phosphates are distinguished from calcium oxalates simply by the presence or absence of P. However, the technique operates independently of the nature of the material; crystalline and amorphous solids are not

13

distinguished. A notable, extensive study of breast tissues was undertaken by Benjamin Galkin[35] who examined discrete tissue deposits from mastectomy specimens. The study surprisingly concluded that many of the smaller deposits did not contain any calcium but a wide range of elements such as silicon and iron. The significance of this work remains unclear and the role of such deposits in calcification development is unknown. However, as a note of caution, due to the high sensitivity of this technique the potential for contamination from specimen processing is high.

A third type of electron microscope examination is the use of electron diffraction. Although specimen preparation is difficult, this method is specific for crystalline phase. However, its application to breast tissue deposits has been very limited. Tornos et al.[36] applied a combination of techniques that included electron diffraction (to a single specimen) from which calcium oxalate monohydrate crystals were identified. A similar, earlier study[37] of a single histopathological section containing crystallites indicated a good crystallographic match to b-HAP.

A technique often used by mineralogists and, in particular, crystallographers studying bone mineral, is that of infrared (IR) spectroscopy. Through the determination of preferential IR absorption bands by bonded atoms, specific molecular species can be identified. This has been previously applied to breast tissue calcifications to demonstrate, in three cases, the presence of calcium oxalate dihydrate[38]. Recently, and increasingly, there has been a more extensive use of IR spectroscopy for examining biological systems, as the analysis probe can be formed within an optical microscope system[39]. Recent work[40] has demonstrated significant differences between the organic components of normal and malignant breast tissues. However, due to the complex nature of the specimens, it is difficult to assign differences to specific changes in the tissue chemistry.

The greatest phase specificity undoubtedly derives from diffraction methods. The most common diffraction probes are X-rays with a wavelength of approximately 0.1 nm, although neutron diffraction is generally also well utilised. However, X-ray diffraction measurements have rarely been performed on breast tissue materials, although they routinely provide definitive phase information within a wide range of fields such as mineralogy, forensic and materials science. Further details are provided in the following section.

In summary, and from a crystallographic perspective, despite the probable significance of phase and microstructural characteristics of deposits forming within biological tissues, there have been very few definitive studies, using appropriate (phase-specific) analytical techniques, of breast calcifications. This has resulted in a common belief, propagated through contemporary literature, that the phases of breast calcifications are well known. The principal sources of evidence upon which this belief is based are summarised in Table 13.2 and comprise 92 patients from a narrow target population. None of the experimental data were collected with sensitive detectors and no analysis beyond phase identification has ever been performed. Further, most of the specimens examined were only representative of "mature" calcification.

X-ray diffraction

X-ray diffraction is a coherent scattering process that occurs when X-ray photons pass through any material. In fact, these scattered photons and the information contained therein are produced during all routine radiological examinations. However, as they do not directly contribute to image formation, they are disregarded. Crystallographically,

Table 13.2 Investigations where phase specific methodologies have been employed to examine breast tissue calcifications

Experimental probe	Recording medium	Specimens	Reference
X-ray diffraction	Film	Three cases, all carcinoma	28
X-ray diffraction	Film	11 patients, malignant and benign	60
X-ray diffraction	Film	49 patients, range of pathologies	43
X-ray diffraction	Film	23 patients, range of pathologies	44
Electron diffraction	Film	One specimen (?), carcinoma	37
Electron diffraction	Film	One specimen, preselected birefringent	36
Infrared spectroscopy	Digital	Three cases (sections), single crystals extracted	38

13

all the structural information is provided by these photons.

For examination of biological minerals there are several key characteristics that can be derived from diffraction data. As is typical of many analytical techniques, X-ray diffraction data from polycrystalline materials may be reduced to a pattern ("diffractogram") containing intensity maxima at specific angular positions, θ, around the specimen (see inset of Fig. 13.2). The angular position of each diffraction maxima is related simply to the interrogating X-ray wavelength, λ, and the perpendicular distance between atomic planes within the sample material, d, through Braggs' Law,

$$\lambda = 2d\sin\theta.$$

The integrated intensities and peak positions are unique for each crystalline phase and thus may be exploited for phase identification. Even when the chemistry is similar, e.g. COD and COM, the diffraction patterns are quite distinct (see Fig. 13.2). Accurate determinations of lattice parameters can be obtained from the peak positions and thus small changes in stoichiometry revealed and quantified. Modern digital technologies (e.g. area or "moving point" detectors) for recording diffraction data have all but replaced film as a recording medium and thus errors from film processing, insensitivity etc. have been significantly reduced.

Microstructural information is inherent within the shape of each diffraction maxima. If crystallite dimensions are less than about 0.2 µm (which is the case for most b-HAP) then the diffraction peaks become broadened in a systematic manner. At these dimensions, optical microscopy and even SEM becomes very limited. Anisotropic broadening between different maxima may be employed to determine average crystallite morphology. A confounding effect, however, is that of small, local variations in lattice parameters (referred to as "microstrain") caused by disordering effects such as stoichiometric gradients, which also broaden the diffraction maxima. A diffraction peak may thus be broadened by finite crystallite size or microstrain, or more likely for biological calcifications a combination of both. For example examine the bone diffraction data presented in Figure 13.2 compared to that of

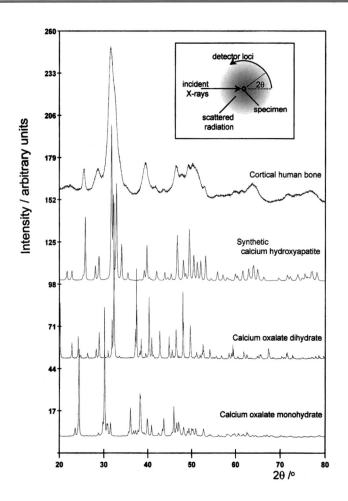

Fig. 13.2
Diffraction data from relevant crystaline phases. Inset shows the conventional X-ray diffraction geometry.

the synthetic calcium hydroxyapatite. The peaks within the bone data are markedly broader than those of the structurally more "perfect", stoichiometric synthetic material. Fortunately, there are several analytical methods that may be applied to diffraction data to separate these effects and provide estimates of crystallite size and microstrain[41].

Diffraction data are also sensitive to the orientation distributions of crystallites with specimens. This is important, for example, in the mechanical functionality of bone that is dependent upon the preferred growth directions of the mineral crystallites.

Finally, the integrated intensities of diffraction peaks contain information concerning the contents of the average unit cell. Thus, by using these data, a complete structural model of the unit cell may be derived and refined. In the case of calcifications it is the model refinement that is of most value, as the structural prototype for b-HAP is well known. The refinement process for polycrystalline materials is commonly known as the Rietveld method and information about precise atomic positions (and therefore distortions) and site occupancies (e.g. Ca deficiencies) may, in principle, be obtained.

Although diffraction analyses are utilised extensively outside the field of medicine, there are limitations in their use applied to biological tissues. Although diffraction is highly phase-specific, with conventional, laboratory X-ray sources, the technique is not highly sensitive and only provides spatial averages. This can lead to ambiguity when analysing homogeneous materials such as b-HAP. With optimum laboratory conditions a phase determination of calcific materials requires at least ~10 µg of material. In the context of breast tissue calcifications, however, the total mass of mineral in, for example, a typical core-cut biopsy specimen, is relatively small and may be dispersed through a relatively large mass of organic tissue. Further, with a small crystallite size and low structural symmetry (resulting in large numbers of diffraction maxima), unambiguous phase identification and microstructural characterisation is challenging, due to significant numbers of overlapping diffraction peaks. Undertaking diffraction experiments using pathological slides is not feasible, due to the limited mass of crystalline material and because the embedding wax (even when apparently removed using xylene) produces a strong diffraction signal masking that of the deposits. However, early work using X-ray diffraction[42,43] examined mammary calcifications removed by microdissection. COD was identified from the diffraction data, although actual specimen numbers and any crystalline HAP identification were not made clear in either of the studies. Further early diffraction data were also collected from dissected deposits and were determined to consist of COD, HAP and amorphous calcium phosphate. However, the distinction between small quantities of truly amorphous and poorly crystalline materials is very difficult. Perhaps the most comprehensive and sensitive X-ray diffraction work to date was that of Fandos-Morera et al.[44]. Using a specialised diffraction camera, Fandos-Morera et al.

examined crystals that had been chemically isolated (aggressively?) from breast tissue. Phases identified were b-HAP, calcium oxalate (hydration state not provided), oxalic acid, calcite and aragonite.

Thus although, in principle, diffraction can provide a large number of mineral characteristics; in practice for biogenic deposits, a great deal of care is required, both in data collection and interpretation. However, it is one of very few, truly phase-specific methodologies and thus one that must be adopted if this information is required. Therefore, recent research has involved the use of specialist radiation sources such as synchrotron radiation described below.

Synchrotron radiation studies

The use of synchrotron radiation (SR) is not widespread in the field of medicine and, in fact, few health care professionals have even heard of it. SR sources provide multiple, extremely intense and tuneable beams of photons over a wide range of energies from IR through to hard X-rays. Its advent has revolutionised many experimental techniques and SR is increasingly being applied across many fields from macroscopic imaging to molecular dynamics. It has spawned several methods for studying live and wet tissue samples yielding information on both structure and composition on all length scales down to atomic resolution. Such techniques have played a crucial role in the development of molecular biology and the solution of protein structures. The application of SR in the field of radiology is now expanding and it is clear that very substantial improvements in image quality and patient dose can be realised.

Although there are currently more than 50 SR sources world-wide (for example, see Fig. 13.3), the use of SR for medical research is still for the most part, in its infancy. The applications of SR to medicine are many and

13

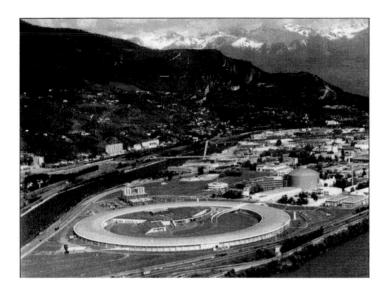

Fig. 13.3
The European Synchroton Radiation Facility sited at Grenoble, France

13

varied. The use of SR sources offers the potential for considerable improvements in some of the techniques already routinely used in medicine, and also makes possible entirely new procedures. Some of these techniques can be applied in vivo, whilst others are more suited to in vitro studies that are therefore potential constituents of the pathologist's tool kit.

The properties of synchrotron radiation can be summarised as follows:

- very high intensity
- a broad and continuous spectrum from infrared to X-rays
- natural collimation
- small source size
- high polarisation
- pulsed time structure.

It is the combination of these properties that makes SR a unique and vastly superior X-ray source than conventional sealed tubes for a very wide range of scientific and technical applications. In particular, the high-intensity, natural collimation and continuous spectrum makes possible the production of intense, tuneable, monochromatic beams of radiation which simply cannot be produced in any other way. The selection of a small wavelength band from the broad white radiation spectrum is achieved by using monochromators fabricated from "perfect" single crystals that exploit Braggs law (see the section on X-ray diffraction).

The traditional and most frequent use of SR has been for X-ray diffraction experiments. These have played a major role in the development of molecular and structural biology, areas that are set to expand further. The human genome project alone is likely to identify in excess of 10 000 proteins, many of which will have to be structurally analysed in order to determine their function. The structure of a protein has a major effect upon its functionality and knowledge of protein sequence is not sufficient to predict its function. Molecules pack in crystals in a non-random manner and are governed by the same rules that apply when the molecule binds to its macromolecular receptor. The results of high-resolution structure analyses based upon X-ray diffraction studies of crystals, provide information that is invaluable for modelling drug–receptor binding. Drug design on the basis of this information is in its infancy, but has accelerated in recent years as a deeper understanding of the required structural principles has begun to emerge.

SR X-ray diffraction is not restricted to the study of crystalline materials but can also yield a wealth of information on fibrous tissues and even solutions, where small and weakly scattering or dilute samples can still produce useful diffracted intensities. Most biological systems have some degree of spatial ordering and SR X-ray diffraction can still be used to provide extremely useful structural information. This type of diffraction is known by the generic term of non-crystalline diffraction, and there are a large number of medically significant projects taking place throughout the world, including studies of protein folding, tubulin assembly and transdermal drug delivery. Specific examples of studies of fibrous biological tissues include examinations of the cornea[45] (which has a stromal region of stacked lamellae, each being composed of a parallel array of collagen fibrils) and muscle[46]. A further example relevant to breast structures is described in greater detail below.

Radiological applications of SR have recently included development of several imaging modalities. These include coronary angiography (including dichromography), bronchography, multiple energy computed tomography, and fluorescent computed tomography. All have been shown to produce high quality images in vivo, with future exploitation expected to provide new insights into diagnosis and disease progression. Radiotherapy applications, exploiting a novel approach using multiple SR microbeam applicators, have shown remarkable results in terms of cellular survivability when compared to conventional methods. Both the imaging and therapeutic applications of SR have been comprehensively reviewed by Lewis[47].

Mammography with SR

Using conventional mammography, lesions of less than 2–3 mm are very difficult to detect. The dedicated mammography X-ray sources are operated at 25–30 kVp. The spectrum from such sealed tubes consists of two fluorescence lines at 17.4 and 19.6 keV superimposed upon a Bremsstrahlung continuum. The characteristic lines themselves represent only 25% of the total flux. Whilst the optimum energy for mammography is known to be in the region of 17–21 keV (it varies slightly with breast thickness and density), the continuum of radiation above 20 keV produces a diffused background in the resulting radiograph that serves only to diminish contrast. It was reported in 1992[48] that tuneable monochromatic SR beams offered the potential to image the breast with higher contrast and perhaps a lower dose than is possible with a conventional mammography set. The basic principle is illustrated in Figure 13.4(a). The monochromaticity of SR results in all the incident photons usefully contributing to the image and the inherent collimation of the beam allows slits to be placed both before and after the breast thereby greatly reducing scatter. The image is constructed by scanning the patient or possibly the beam.

The first tests on phantoms and excised breast tissue, performed at the Adone SR source in Frascati[49], demonstrated that images of higher contrast could be recorded with a similar or lower dose than on a conventional mammography set. Subsequent work with phantoms[50] has shown that 20-keV SR images have comparable contrast to those obtained in conventional mammograms but with a skin dose that is 10 times smaller. At 17 keV, substantially higher contrast is obtained with less than half the skin dose for a conventional mammogram. Our work on the UK's SR source at Daresbury has recently confirmed these results[51]. To fully

13

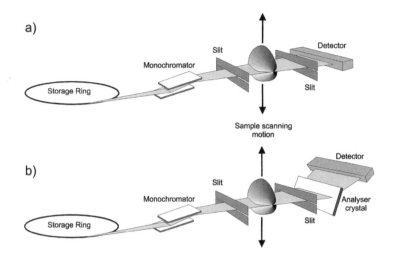

a)

Detector

Slit

Monochromator

Slit

Storage Ring

Sample scanning
motion

b)

Detector

Slit

Slit

Monochromator

Analyser
crystal

Storage Ring

Slit

Fig. 13.4
Mammography using Synchroton radiation. Both of the systems illustrated utilise a tuneable monochromatic beam and slits to reject scattered radiation. In (b) an analyser crystal is used to enhance scatter rejection and improve contrast.

13

establish the potential of this technique, a dedicated mammography beamline is being built on the "ELETTRA" SR machine at Sincrotrone Trieste, Italy[52].

A very exciting recent development is the latest work at the National Synchrotron Light Source (USA). Termed diffraction-enhanced imaging (DEI), a second analyser crystal is placed after the breast tissue which then transmits only those photons having a specific energy (see Fig. 13.4b). Not only does this system have excellent scatter rejection, it has been used to produce some quite spectacular contrast enhancements by using the analyser to select those photons which have been very slightly deviated from the beam[53].

It has been demonstrated that with SR, and particularly DEI, greatly improved spatial and contrast resolution can be achieved and thus there is the potential to detect and characterise calcifications during mammography. This may therefore result in higher sensitivity and specificity for diagnosis, based upon appearance rather than simply distribution of the calcifications.

Breast tissue collagen organisation

In a current research programme at the Daresbury SR source, breast tissue samples are being studied by X-ray diffraction. It is hoped that the work will determine whether differences at the molecular level, in the tissue surrounding tumours, can be observed by diffraction techniques. Work is concentrating on collagen structure, calcifications and adipose tissue. Recently we have been examining collagen structures within breast tissues using small angle X-ray scattering (SAXS) to characterise collagen's supramolecular ordering. The rationale for this work is based upon observations that breast tumours display aberrant collagen organisation in the tumour stroma[54,55]. Furthermore, extensive alteration of the extracellular matrix has been observed in invasive colorectal carcinomas where the collagen derangement is attributed to both enzymatic degradation and altered neosynthesis.

Our results thus far have demonstrated that highly significant differences can be

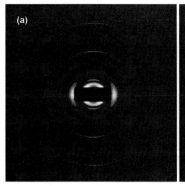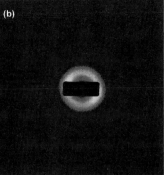

Fig. 13.5
2-dimensional, small angle X-ray scattering distributions from breast tissue core-cut biopsy specimens of (a) normal tissues and, (b) malignant tumour tissue. Note the lack of well defined diffraction maxima in (b) indicating the loss of ultrastructural order. The dark rectangular central region is a lead absorber to stop the direct beam reaching the detector.

detected in the collagen order and atomic spacings of normal, malignant and benign breast tissues[56].

Perhaps, more importantly, it appears that these differences are detectable several centimetres away from the lesion. An example of the SAXS data is presented in Figure 13.5, which illustrates the marked difference between normal and malignant breast tissues. We are currently pursuing further work involving larger patient numbers and a wider range of tumour types.

Crystalline materials within breast tissues

The difficulty in describing the crystallographic details of breast tissue calcification is that they are simply unknown. The real significance and formation mechanisms of breast calcifications are also unknown although it has been suggested that the difference between lamellar and granular architectures is due to calcium precipitation in either proteinaceous or cellular environments respectively[16]. Thus only a brief outline of current evidence is provided below. There are probably a number of different formation mechanisms in breast tissues, some passive (related to necrosis) and some active. These inevitably produce a range of phases and mineral stoichiometries.

Generally, formation processes and models have been inferred from the location of the calcifications within tissues rather than tissue chemistry and calcification crystallography. Perhaps the most fundamental (and, on the whole, currently lacking) crystallographic information is simply the phase of material being formed.

Specific interest in the crystalline phases forming within breast tissues has previously arisen, principally due to:

1. Understanding discrepancies between radio-opacities seen on mammograms and those observed during histopathology. This has been ascribed partly due to difficulties observing what is assumed to be COD in biopsy specimens (normal histopathological stains are ineffective) and its apparent preferential loss during sectioning[57].

2. Assessment of the diagnostic value of crystalline phase. It is often assumed that breast calcification phase is either (i) calcium oxalate dihydrate, formed perhaps as a result of secretory activity of epithelial cells[58] and/or neoplasia, or (ii) dystrophic calcium hydroxyapatite[59]. However, careful examination of the definitive evidence (i.e. phase-specific) upon which this assumption is founded (see Table 13.2) reveals several unsatisfactory features of

13

the data. These include very small specimen numbers, confounding specimen preparation methods and highly selective tissue types (only very mature/large deposits have thus far been studied).

The association of calcium oxalates with benign disease or LCIS is in contrast to an association of b-HAP with both benign and infiltrating carcinomas.[60] Thus some diagnostic value may be directly attributable to phase. However, the detailed diffraction work of Fandos-Morera[44] did not coincide with this generally held view. Perhaps a further difficulty here is the complete lack of any genuine "control" data arising from non-diseased breast tissues.

3. Examining the effects of silicone prosthetic devices to determine the likelihood of silicate deposition and toxicity of silicon based minerals[31,61].

The b-HAP of breast tissues is undoubtedly non-stoichiometric and it is highly likely that the "amorphous calcium phosphate" often referred to within current literature is actually crystalline b-HAP. It is probably the most frequently observed calcific phase within breast tissues, where it may appear as opaque, basophilic deposits with small crystallite size. It has also been referred to[59] as a "type II" calcification and exclusively (probably mistakenly) associated with infiltrating carcinoma[61]. It has been suggested that b-HAP is the result of any pathological alteration of breast tissue, whereas the formation of other phases may suggest a specific tissue change.

In contrast, calcium oxalate dihydrate (mineral name "weddellite"), probably tends to form relatively large polyhedral and birefringent crystallites. It has been referred to as "type I" calcifications and its presence has been associated with lobular carcinoma in situ or benign lesions (including apocrine metaplasia). Although its most common formation route is through oxalic acid, this is rarely observed to crystallise in breast tissues. This, of course, may be a consequence of the non-phase-specific analytical techniques employed.

Although calcium oxalate dihydrate is an end point of metabolism (there are no oxalate degenerative enzymes in humans), oxalate resorption has been demonstrated in renal and postmortem thyroid tissues[62]. Any such resorption would inevitably result in tissue changes in response to the liberation of toxic oxalate ions. Calcium oxalate dihydrate is more unstable thermodynamically than the monohydrate phase. In other biosystems, COD has been shown to convert to the monohydrate forms unless stabilised[63]. Perhaps surprisingly, calcium oxalate monohydrate is rarely reported to be found within breast tissues. Within the thyroid it has been suggested that examination of (what is assumed to be) COD, features may indicate the functional state of lesions[64]. Within occular tissues, dystrophic oxalosis has been ascribed to the presence of intraocular ascorbic acid[65] and activity of the retinal pigment epithelium[66].

Through a careful examination of previous investigations, there would appear to be some evidence for a range of phases formed within breast tissues. These are listed in Table 13.3. The majority of these are not regularly reported, due to the low specificity of the methods routinely employed to examine breast tissues and, perhaps, destructive specimen processing techniques. If indeed there is a wide range of crystalline phases being formed then undoubtedly specific crystallisation mechanisms are responsible.

Formation mechanisms

For any physiologic or pathologic crystal deposition, a sequence of fundamental events involving tissue changes must occur. These include a local increase in ionic

Table 13.3 Phases reportedly identified within breast tissues

Chemical name	Chemical formula	Mineral name	Reference
Calcium hydroxyapatite	$Ca_5(PO_4)_3(OH)$[1]	Dahllite	60
Calcium oxalate dihydrate	$Ca(CO_2)_2 2H_2O$	Weddellite	60
Calcium oxalate monohydrate	$Ca(CO_2)_2 2H_2O$	Whewellite	36
Calcium oxalate	$Ca(CO_2)_2$	–	44
Calcium carbonate	$CaCO_3$	Calcite	44
Calcium carbonate	$CaCO_3$	Aragonite	44
Oxalic acid	$C_2H_2O_4$	–	44
Tricalcium phosphate	$Ca_3(PO_4)_2$	Whitlockite	28
Amorphous CAP	Ca_xP_y	–	60

[1] Refers to b-HAP, dahllite being carbonate substituted HAP. Where multiple reference sources are available (e.g. in cases when b-HAP is reported), only one is provided.

13

species, a change in pH and the formation of a deposition nucleator or promoter[68]. The nature of these events in breast tissue has not been established. Pathologic b-HAP is often correlated with the presence of membrane debris such as that found associated with cell necrosis. However, in many studies the cause–effect direction has not been established; studies have been unable to determine if crystals cause necrosis or necrotic tissue facilitates crystal growth[67]. Further, within breast tissues, many of the crystalline deposits, particularly formed from relatively small crystallites, are not associated with areas of necrosis, although a characteristic of all necrotic breast tissue is that it absorbs calcium.

The apparent similarity between the b-HAP formed within breast and that of osteo tissues, has prompted several studies examining common features of the formation mechanisms. However, calcific phase deposition in breast tissues is unlike "normal" ossification, as breast calcification is not uniquely associated with collagen and, in any case, the collagen of breast carcinoma tissues does not possess the structural order required to support ossification[68,69].

Nonetheless, several bone matrix proteins have been identified at raised concentrations in malignant lesions and calcified tissues. Macrophages rather than tumour cells, that have been shown to express osteopontin[70] (this has a high binding affinity for HA), have also been associated with necrotic areas of breast tumours, although this is not unique to breast tissues[71]. Further, it has been recently demonstrated[72] that breast cancer cells express bone sialoprotein (normally associated with bone mineralisation and remodelling) and this may be used as a potential indicator of the ability of the cells to metastasise to bone. An early stage marker for this is likely to be calcification. Intriguingly, it has also been suggested that such bone matrix proteins, produced by breast cells, may further be responsible for the high osteotropism of breast cancer cells and a molecular basis for this, based upon interactions between metastatic cancer cells and osteoclasts, has recently been proposed[73].

Other indicators of specific formation mechanisms that involve active protein participation may be derived from elemental analyses of specimens; many enzymes require metallorganic cofactors. Such studies have shown that several elements, including Mg and Zn[74], are significantly elevated within cancerous tissues. It is well known that Mg has an inhibiting effect on the conversion of amorphous calcium phosphate to hydroxyapatite. Other elements such as silicon may also be implicated in specific formation mechanisms.[75]

Another facet to breast tissue–calcification interactions has been developed through the careful examination of calcium phosphate crystallites associated with osteoarthritic joint disease. Here a clear link between the presence of basic calcium phosphate crystals (these include b-HAP, octacalcium phosphate and tricalcium phosphate) and the degree of cartilage degeneration has been established[76]. The causal nature of this link has been shown to be probably due to the apparent ability of b-HAP crystallites to induce mitogenesis and secretion of matrix metalloproteases[77,78]. It has also been demonstrated that human articular cartilage matrix vesicles can be stimulated to produce crystalline calcium pyrophosphate dihydrate if exposed to adenosine triphosphate (ATP) and b-HAP crystals without ATP[79,80]. Recently, a genetic basis for control of tissue calcification through regulation of cellular pyrophosphate levels in a mouse model has been postulated[81]. The consequences of these recent findings for calcification of breast tissues are unclear. No pyrophosphate phase has ever been reported observed within breast tissues.

In summary, breast tissue is a complex, dynamic chemical environment that, in principle, enables the formation and resorption of a range of inorganic crystalline deposits. It is clear that currently there are no satisfactory mechanistic models for the formation of breast tissue calcifications and no definitive data relating the deposition of specific inorganic phases to the aetiology and development of breast disease. There is, however,

a growing body of circumstantial evidence that may form the basis of such a model and there is certainly a central role to be played by the calcification ultrastructure within any such model.

Work in progress

The crystallography of breast tissue calcifications is important (a) to assess the diagnostic and prognostic potential of the calcific structures and (b) to help map the natural history of disease processes, through premalignant, cancerous and metastatic stages. In selecting appropriate data collection and analysis techniques, both specificity and sensitivity need to be assessed. Ideally the calcifications should be examined within the tissues in order to retain any spatial relationship between them. Thus, correlation and corroboration with histopathological data would be possible. We are unaware of any such studies that have been performed and even the detail that arises from diffractometer experiments is rarely, if ever, reported.

Our recent work has involved diffraction characterisation of a range of breast tissues. We have used small angle diffraction to study changes to collagen with malignancy (see previous section) and wide angle diffraction to study the nature of calcifications. Although not yet attempted with breast tissues, in principle, these two measurement regimens may be combined into a single experiment.

Our diffraction studies of calcifications have included the examination of both dissected crystalline masses and core-cut biopsy specimens containing crystallite populations. The dissected samples were studied in the laboratory using conventional powder diffraction measuring facilities. The b-HAP data from breast tissue deposits (see Fig. 13.6b) was subsequently compared to that from other biogenic calcifications (bone, ureteric calculi and aortic medial calcification) using

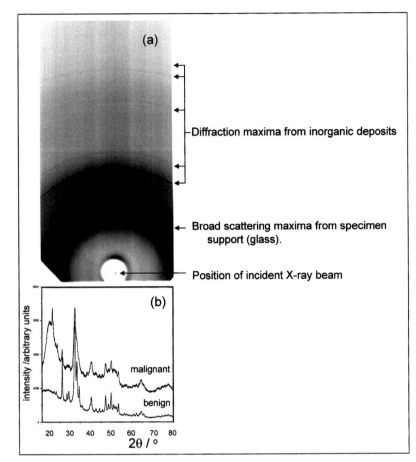

(a)

Diffraction maxima from inorganic deposits

Broad scattering maxima from specimen support (glass).

Position of incident X-ray beam

(b)

malignant

benign

intensity /arbitrary units

20 30 40 50 60 70 80
2θ / °

13

Fig. 13.6
Diffraction data from core-cut biopsy specimens.
(a) section of 2-D intensity using synchrotron radiation,
(b) 1-D data from large, dissected deposits.

the Rietveld refinement method. Although specimen numbers were limited, it was apparent that the breast calcification was something of an extreme mineral, possessing the greatest lattice parameter (along the c-axis) and smallest crystallite size[82]. The full significance of this will be realised as further data become available. However, it may be related to differences in the initial deposition mechanisms. Further preliminary work (as yet unreported) employing synchrotron radiation examined, for the first time, core-cut biopsy specimens. Utilising a small (0.5 × 0.5 mm) incident X-ray beam, each unfixed specimen was oscillated through the beam,

ensuring complete illumination during 30-minute data collections. An image plate recorded the diffraction data (see Fig. 13.6a), which was subsequently reduced to one-dimension by radial integration. A phase-matching routine indicated the presence of b-HAP and other, as yet unidentified crystalline materials that do not appear to correspond to those within Table 13.3.

We hope in future to undertake more extensive studies on similar specimens, and produce a complete account of the calcific phases formed and their crystallographic detail. In vivo characterisation may, to some extent, be developed from emerging technologies such as diffraction-enhanced imaging (see previous section) and/or absorption edge-enhanced imaging (the linear absorption coefficient of HAP is almost three times that of COD at 20 keV). Thus the full diagnostic potential of breast calcifications would be exploited. Naturally, this is critically dependent upon demonstration of the clinical significance of calcification crystallography.

References

1. Piattella L, Zamponi N, Cardinali C, Porfiri L, Tavoni M. Endocranial calcifications, infantile celiac disease, and epilepsy. Childs Nervous System 1993; 9: 172–5.
2. Brown K, Mund DF, Aberle DR, Batra P, Young DA. Intrathoracic calcifications: radiographic features and differential diagnoses. Radiographics 1994; 14: 1247–61.
3. Rieber A. Das fibrolamellare Karzinom. Zeitschrift Gastroenterol 1994; 32: 651–3.
4 Kragel PJ, Aquino MO, Fiorella R, Chapman J. Clinical, radiological and pathological features of medial calcific sclerosis in the breast. Southern Med J 1997; 90: 518–21.
5 McCarty DJ, Lehr JR, Halverson PB. Crystal populations in human synovial fluid; identification of apatite, octacalcium phosphate and tricalcium phosphate. Arthritis Rheum 1983; 26: 1220–4.
6. Mustafina ZhG, D'iakova GA, Galimova RZ, Karzhaubaeva GG. Pathological mineralization in retinoblastoma. Vestnik Oftalmologii 1992; 108: 37–8.
7. Sperrin MW, Rogers KD. The architecture and composition of uroliths. Br J Urol 1998; 82: 781–4.
8. Price JL, Gibbs NM. The relationship between microcalcification and in situ carcinoma of the breast. Clin Radiol 1978; 29: 447–52.
9. Egan RL, McSweeney MB, Sewell CW. Intramammary calcifications without an associated mass in benign and malignant diseases. Radiology 1980; 137: 1–7.
10. Galkin BM, Feig SA, Frasca P, Muir HD, Soriano RZ. Photomicrographs of breast calcifications: correlation with histopathologic diagnosis. Radiographics 1983; 3: 450–77.
11. Kragel PJ, Aquino MO, Fiorella R, Chapman J. Clinical, radiographic and pathologic features of medial calcific sclerosis in the breast. Southern Med J 1997; 90: 518–21.
12. Frouge C, Meunier M, Guinebretiere J-M et al. Polyhedral microcalcifications at mammography: histologic correlation with calcium oxalate. Radiology 1993; 186; 681–4.
13. Holme TC, Reis MM, Thompson A, Robertson A et al. Is mammographic microcalcification of biological significance? Eur J Surg Oncol 1993; 19: 250–3.
14. Albertyn LE. Mammographically indeterminate microcalcifications: can we do any better? Australasia Radiol 1991; 35: 350–7.
15. Stomper PC, Connolly JL. Ductal carcinoma in situ of the breast: correlation between mammographic calcification and tumor subtype. Am J Roentgenol 1992; 159: 483–5.
16. Foschini MP, Fornelli A, Peterse JL, Mignani S, Eusebi V. Microcalcifications in ductal carcinoma in situ of the breast: histochemical and immunohistochemical study. Hum Pathol 1996; 27: 178–83.
17. Tsuchiya A, Kanno M, Hara K, Kimijima I, Abe R. The evaluation of mammographic microcalcification as biological malignancy in breast cancer. Fukushima J Med Sci 1996; 1: 17–22.
18. Tabar L, Chen H, Duffy SW, Yen MF, Chiang CF, Dean PB, Smith RA. A novel method for prediction of long-term outcome of women with T1a, T1b, and 10–14 mm invasive cancers: a prospective study. Lancet 2000; 355: 429–33.
19. Wheeler EJ, Lewis D. An X-ray study of the paracrystalline nature of bone apatite. Calcified Tissue Res 1977; 24: 243–8.
20. Morgan H, Wilson RM, Elliott JC, Dowker SEP, Abderson P. Preparation and characterisation of monoclinic hydroxyapatite and its precipitated carbonate apatite intermediate. Biomaterials 2000; 21: 617–27.
21. Handschin RG, Stern WB. X-ray diffraction studies on the lattice perfection of human bone apatite (Crista Iliaca). Bone 1995; 16: 355S–63S.
22. Wilson RM, Elliott JC, Dowker SEP. Rietveld refinement of the crystallographic structure of human dental enamel apatites. Am Minerol 1999; 84: 1406–14.
23. Fujisawa R, Kuboki Y. Preferential adsorption of dentin and bone acidic proteins on the (100) face of hydroxyapatite crystals. Biochim Biophys Acta 1991; 1075: 56–60.
24. LeGeros RZ, Kijkowska R, Bautista C, LeGeros JP. Synergistic effects of magnesium and carbonate on properties of biological and synthetic apatites. Connective Tissue Res 1995; 33: 203–9.
25. Prudhommeaux F, Schiltz C, Liote F et al. Variation in the inflammatory properties of basic calcium phosphate crystals according to crystal type. Arthritis Rheum 1996; 39: 1319–26.
26. Wiessner JH, Mandel GS, Halverson PB, Mandel NS. The effect of hydroxyapatite crystallinity on hemolysis. Calcified Tissue Intl 1988; 42: 210–19.
27. Osborne CA, Davis LS, Sanne J, Unger LK, O'Brien TD, Clinton CW, Davenport MP. Identification and interpretation of crystalluria in domestic animals: a

light and scanning electron microscopic study. Vet Med 1990; 85: 18–37.

28. Hassler O. Microradiographic investigations of calcifications of the female breast. Cancer 1969; 23: 1103–9.

29. Daculsi G, Bouler J-M, LeGeros RZ. Adaptive crystal formation in normal and pathological calcifications in synthetic calcium phosphate and related biomaterials. Intl Rev Cytol 1997; 172: 129–91.

30. Moritz JD, Luftner Nagel S, Westerhof JP, Oestmann JW, Grabbe E. Microcalcifications in breast core biopsy specimens: disappearance at radiography after storage in formaldehyde. Radiology 1996; 200: 361–3.

31. Pasteris JD, Wopenka B, Freeman JJ, Leroy Young V, Brandon HJ. Medical mineralogy as a new challenge to the geologist: silicates in human mammary tissue? Am Mineral 1999; 84: 997–1008.

32. Terzakis JA. Detection of calcifications in breast biopsies by scanning electron microscopy. Ultrastr Pathol 1998; 22: 181–4.

33. Mihaescu A, Burri G. Calcium oxalate crystals in benign breast cyst fluid. Diagn Cytopathol 1995; 12: 67–70.

34. Torell JA, Knight JP, Marcus PB. Intraluminal calcium hydroxyapatite crystals in breast carcinoma: an ultrastructural study. Ultrastr Pathol 1984; 6: 9–14.

35. Galkin BJ, Frasca P, Feig SA, Holderness KE. Non-calcified breast particles. A possible new marker of breast cancer. Invest Radiol 1982; 17: 119–28.

36. Tornos C, Silva E, El-Nagger A, Pritzker KPH. Calcium oxalate crystals in breast biopsies. The missing calcifications. Am J Surg Pathol 1990; 14: 961–8.

37. Ahmed A. Calcification in human breast carcinomas: ultrastructural observations. J Pathol 1975; 117: 247–51.

38. Going JJ, Anderson TJ, Crocker PR, Levison DA. Weddellite calcification in the breast: 18 cases with implications for breast cancer screening. Histopathology 1990; 16: 119–24.

39. Estepa-Maurice L, Hennequin C, Marfisi C, Bader C, Lacour B, Daudon M. Fourier transform infrared microscopy identification of crystal deposits in tissues. Clin Chem 1996; 105: 576–82.

40. Jackson M, Mansfield JR, Dolenko B, Somorjai RL, Mantsh HH, Watson PH. Classification of breast tumours by grade and steroid receptor status using pattern recognition analysis of infrared spectra. Cancer Detect Prevent 1999; 23: 245–53.

41. Delhez R, deKeijser TH, Langford JI, Louer D, Mittemeijer EJ, Sonneveld EJ. Crystal imperfection broadening and peak shape in the Rietveld method. In: Young RA, Ed. The Rietveld Method. USA, IUCr–Oxford University Press, 1993.

42. Frappart L, Remy I, Lin HC, Bremond A, Raudrant D, Grousson B, Vauzelle JL. Different types of microcalcifications observed in breast pathology: correlations with histopathological diagnosis and radiological examination of operative specimens. Virchows Arch A 1986; 410: 179–87.

43. Frappart L, Boudeulle M, Boumendil J et al. Structure and composition of microcalcifications in benign and malignant lesions of the breast: study by light microscopy, transmission and scanning electron microscopy, microprobe analysis and X-ray diffraction. Hum Pathol 1984; 15: 880–9.

44. Fandos-Morera A, Prats-Esteve M, Tura-Soteras JM, Traveria-Cros A. Breast tumours: composition of microcalcifications. Radiology 1988; 169: 325–7.

45. Meek KM, Blamires T, Elliot GF, Gyi TJ, Nave C. The organisation of collagen fibrils in the human corneal stroma: a synchrotron radiation x-ray diffraction study. Curr Eye Res 1987; 6: 841–6.

46. Lombardi V, Piazzesi G, Ferenczi M, Thirlwell H, Dobbie I, Irving M. Elastic distortion of myosin heads and repriming of the working stroke in muscle. Nature 1995; 374: 553–5.

47. Lewis RA. Medical applications of synchrotron radiation X-rays. Physics Med Biol 1997; 42: 1213–43.

48. Burattini E, Gambaccini M, Marziani M et al. X-ray mammography with synchrotron radiation. Rev Sci Instrum 1992; 63; 638–40.

49. Burattini E, Cossu E, Di Maggio C et al. Mammography with synchrotron radiation. Radiology 1995; 195: 239–44.

50. Johnston RE, Washburn D, Pisano E et al. Preliminary experience with monoenergetic photon mammography. SPIE 1995; 2432: 434–41.

51. Lewis RA, Hufton AP, Hall CJ, Helsby WI, Towns-Andrews E, Slawson S, Boggis CRM. Improvements in image quality and radiation dose in breast imaging. Synchrotron Radiation News 1999; 12: 7–14.

52. Arfelli F, Bravin A, Barbiellini G et al. Digital mammography with synchrotron radiation. Rev Sci Instrum 1995; 66: 1325–8.

53. Zhong Z, Thomlinson W, Chapman D, Sayers D. Implementation of diffraction-enhanced imaging experiments: at the NSLS and APS. Nucl Instrum Methods Physics Res 2000; A450: 556–67.

54. Schonermark MP, Bock O, Buchner A, Steinmeier R, Benbow U, Lenarz T. Quantification of tumor cell invasion using confocal laser scan microscopy. Nat Med 1997; 3: 1167–71.

55. Kauppila S, Stenbäck F, Risteli J, Jukkola A, Risteli L. Aberrant type I and type III collagen gene expression in human breast cancer in vivo. J Pathol 1998; 186: 262–8.

56. Lewis RA, Rogers KD, Hall CJ et al. Breast cancer diagnosis using scattered X-rays. J Synchrotron Radiat 2000; 7: 348–52.

13

57. D'Orsi CJ, Reale FR, Davis MA, Brown VJ. Is calcium oxalate an adequate explanation for nonvisualization of breast specimen calcifications? Radiology 1992; 182: 801–3.

58. Edmundo J, Gonzalez G, Caldwell R, Valaitis J. Calcium oxalate crystals in the breast. Pathology and significance. Am J Surg Pathol 1991; 15: 586–91.

59. Radi MJ. Calcium oxalate crystals in breast biopsies. An overlooked form of microcalcification associated with benign breast disease. Arch Pathol Lab Med 1989; 113: 1367–9.

60. Busing CM, Keppler U, Menges V. Differences in microcalcification in breast tumors. Virchows Archiv A 1981; 393: 307–13.

61. Bellahcene A, Castronovo V. Increased expression of osteonectin and osteopontin, two bone matrix proteins, in human breast cancer. Am J Pathol 1995; 146: 95–100.

62. Bergstrand A, Collste LG, Franksson C et al. Oxalosis in renal transplants following methoxyflurane anaesthesia. Br J Anaesth 1972; 44; 569–74.

63. Rogers KD, Sperrin MW, MacLean EJ. A synchrotron study of bladder urolith architecture. Powder Diffraction 2000; 15: 94–100.

64. Katoh R, Kawaoi A, Muramatsu A, Hemmi A, Suzuki K. Birefringent (calcium oxalate) crystals in thyroid diseases – a clinicopathological study with possible implications for differential diagnosis. Am J Surg Pathol 1993; 17: 698–705.

65. Gardner A. Retinal oxalosis. Br J Ophthalmol 1974; 58: 613–19.

66. Jensen OA. Calcium oxalate crystals localised in the eye. Acta Ophthalmol 1975; 53: 187–96.

67. Boskey AL, Bullough PG, Vigorita V, DiCarlo E. Calcium–acidic phospholipid–phosphate complexes in human hydroxyapatite-containing pathologic deposits. Am J Pathol 1988; 133: 22–9.

68. Rogers KD, Lewis RA, Hall CJ et al. Preliminary observations of breast tumor collagen. Synchrotron Radiation News 1999; 12; 15–20.

69. Pucci-Minafra I, Luparello C, Andriolo M, Basirico L, Aquino A, Minafra S. A new form of tumor and fetal collagen that binds laminin. Biochemistry 1993; 32: 7421–7.

70. Hirota S, Ito A, Nagoshi J et al. Expression of bone matrix protein messenger ribonucleic acids in human breast cancers. Lab Invest 1995; 72: 64–9.

71. Brown LF, Papadopoulos-Sergiou A, Berse B et al. Osteopontin expression and distribution in human carcinomas. Am J Pathol 1994; 145: 610–23.

72. Bellahcene A, Castronovo V. Expression of bone matrix proteins in human breast cancer: potential roles in microcalcification formation and in the genesis of bone metastases. Bull Cancer 1997; 84: 17–24.

73. Yoneda T. Cellular and molecular basis of preferential metastasis of breast cancer to bone. J Orthopaed Sci 2000; 5: 75–81.

74. Santoliquido PM, Southwick HW, Olwin JH. Trace metal levels in cancer of the breast. Surg Gynecol Obstet 1976; 142: 65–70.

75. Carlisle EM. Silicon. Biochem Essent Ultratrace Elements 1984; 3: 257–91.

76. Halverson PB, McCarty DJ. Patterns of radiographic abnormalities associated with basic calcium phosphate and calcium pyrophosphate crystal deposition in the knee. Annu Rheum Dis 1986; 45: 603–5.

77. Cheung HS, Story MT, McCarty DJ. Mitogenic effects of hydroxyapatite and calcium pyrophosphate dihydrate crystals on cultured mammalian cells. Arthritis Rheum 1984; 27: 668–74.

78. McCarthy GM, Mitchell PG, Struve JS, Cheung HS. Basic calcium phosphate crystals cause co-ordinate induction and secretion of collagenase and stromelysin. J Cell Physiol 1992; 153: 140–6.

79. Derfus BA, Kurtin SM, Camacho NP, Kurup I, Ryan LM. Comparison of matrix vesicles derived from normal and osteoarthritic human articular cartilage. Connective Tissue Res 1996; 35: 337–42.

80. Derfus BA, Kranendonk S, Camacho NP, Mandel N, Kushnaryov V, Lynch K, Ryan LM. Human osteoarthritic cartilage matrix vesicles generate both calcium pyrophosphate dihydrate and apatite in vitro. Calcified Tissue Intl 1998; 63: 258–62.

81. Ho AM, Johnson MD, Kingsley DM. Role of the mouse ank gene in control of tissue calcification and arthritis. Science 2000; 289: 265–70.

82. Rogers KD. Initial Rietveld characterisation of biological calcifications. Powder Diffraction 1997; 12: 175–9.

Index